AUTO

Activate Your Natural Self-Cleansing Process to Lose Weight, Reduce Inflammation, Boost Energy and Live Longer Through Intermittent Fasting, Keto Diet, Exercise and Other Methods

© **Jaida Ellison**

© **Text Copyright 2019 by Jaida Ellison**

All rights reserved. No part of this guide may be reproduced in any form without permission in writing from the publisher except in the case of brief quotations embodied in critical articles or reviews and certain other noncommercial uses permitted by copyright law.

Legal & Disclaimer

The information contained in this book and its contents are not designed to replace or take the place of any form of medical or professional advice and are not meant to replace the need for independent medical, financial, legal or other professional advice or services, as may be required. The content and information in this book have been provided for educational and entertainment purposes only.

The content and information contained in this book has been compiled from sources deemed reliable, and it is accurate to the best of the Author's knowledge, information and belief. However, the Author cannot guarantee its accuracy and validity and cannot be held liable for any errors and/or omissions. Furthermore, changes are periodically made to this book as and when needed. Where appropriate and/or necessary, you must consult a professional (including but not limited to your doctor, attorney, financial advisor or such other professional advisor) before using any of the suggested remedies, techniques, or information in this book.

Upon using the contents and information contained in this book, you agree to hold harmless the Author from and against any damages, costs, and expenses, including any legal fees potentially resulting from the application of any of the information provided by this book. This disclaimer applies to any loss, damages or injury caused by the use and application, whether directly or indirectly, of any advice or information presented, whether for breach of contract, tort, negligence, personal injury, criminal intent, or under any other cause of action.

You agree to accept all risks of using the information presented inside this book.

You agree that by continuing to read this book, where appropriate and/or necessary, you shall consult a professional before using any of the suggested remedies, techniques, or information in this book.

TABLE OF CONTENTS

FOREWORD.. 1

INTRODUCTION 3

CHAPTER ONE 8

   What is Autophagy? 8

   Basic terminologies... 10

   Types of autophagy 13

   The mechanisms behind autophagy 15

   Autophagic regulators 18

CHAPTER TWO: How To Achieve Autophagy............... 22

   Keto diet.. 22

   Fasting... 24

   Exercise... 34

   Dietary tips 38

   Other methods to induce autophagy 43

CHAPTER THREE.. 50

   Autophagy in weight loss.. 50

   Autophagy in Metabolic Diseases 54

CHAPTER FOUR: Autophagy in Neurodegenerative Disorders... 63

   Parkinson's disease... 65

   Alzheimer's disease 71

   Prion disease 80

   Amyotrophic Lateral Sclerosis (ALS) 82

CHAPTER FIVE 86
How autophagy helps you build a stronger immune system 86
Autophagy and HIV 101
Autophagy and Tuberculosis 121
CHAPTER SIX 131
Autophagy and Cancer 131
Stay young forever through autophagy 141
CHAPTER SEVEN: Autophagic Lifestyle 146
Autophagic meal plan 146
Meals that help you achieve autophagy 158
CONCLUSION 206

FOREWORD

This book is a full package of everything you need to know about autophagy. It gives very important details about this emerging concept in a casual relaxed tone. The reader grasps life-saving tips and knowledge, without even knowing. The vocabulary and language used are basic and do not require expertise or prior knowledge to understand.

This book enables the reader to understand more about autophagy, its types, mechanisms and how it affects the body (short and long-term benefits), ways of implementing it and most importantly how to live an autophagy-based lifestyle.

This book helps the reader retrace his or her steps, especially as pertains to food (eating *healthy*). Longman dictionary describes food as a material consisting essentially of proteins, carbohydrates and fat that is taken in by living things and supplies energy and sustains processes (e.g. growth as well as repair) necessary for survival. This definition shows how far we have deviated from the principal purpose of eating, considered to be both to nourish and sustain our life. Exercising is not left out. Autophagy basically talks about living healthy.

Each chapter in this book is a gold mine. There is always something new and fascinating, separately conveying and driving home their respective points. Therefore, even if you decide to pick chapters randomly, a lot of knowledge and information will still be gained.

Autophagy is discussed in phases designed progressively to increase assimilation. Firstly, a brief rundown of autophagy is given, followed by more exciting details.

INTRODUCTION

Nowadays, every step taken in our world revolves around technological efficiency. More efficient cars are being built. They are faster, more advanced, and most importantly, they are made to consume less energy (e.g. fuel, diesel, etc.). Today, cars that can use water, electricity and many other cleaner sources of energy are being manufactured and marketed around the globe. This drive for improved efficiency is not limited to cars alone. It applies to almost every other thing (or technology) in the world today. Our bodies are no different. Scientists and researchers, medical practitioners, nutritionists and many more professionals around the world work around the clock to improve the efficiency of the human body. The purpose of their work can be summarized in one sentence: improve the quality of human life, reduce mortality, and increase human longevity.

Living a healthy and fulfilling life doesn't happen by merely wishing it. Without a doubt, some people are naturally stronger than others. For some reason, most likely genetics, their bodies are more robust (able to withstand more). This cannot change the fact that living healthy will prolong the quality of your life. Not just the quality, but its length too.

Over the years, many lifestyles have been adopted to achieve these targets (longevity). Examples include vegan lifestyles, exercise-based living, etc., all with the same intent: to improve the quality of life and increase longevity.

Let's introduce autophagy, shall we! Autophagy can be described as a combination of all these healthy lifestyles. Autophagy refreshes, enhances and boosts the body in a way never before seen. This is a *book of life.* It is bound to affect your life positively. Why? The answer is simple and straightforward.

We all want to live longer! This is something we all want.

To live a life free from sickness, pain and discomfort. Although this book focuses on autophagy, an emerging health concept, it is a must-read for everyone, both young and old. This is not a law book that only educates the reader on the dos and don'ts of autophagy and how to achieve it. It is practically oriented and offers endless resources on the subject. To cap it all, details on autophagy and the ways to achieve it are provided in a completely new way.

Maintaining a healthy lifestyle cannot be overemphasized. Recent statistics have highlighted that disease occurrence is more than ever on the increase (number of people affected by disease). A new case study has shown that over one fifth of the world's population was afflicted by diverse diseases. The most insane thing is the fact that millions of people are diagnosed with diseases every day. Further statistics show that every second, thousands of people are dying from a disease. Astonishingly, scientists predict that these statistics will go up.

What makes autophagy intriguing is the fact that it is rooted in most parts of our everyday lives. This includes how and what we eat, the quantity of food we consume, daily routines, working out and much more. Simply put, living healthy stems from our lifestyle. Unhealthy foods are the cliché while exercising is now seen as a luxury. Although medications, exercise and adequate rest all contribute to a good management and treatment of illnesses, the role of a proper and healthy lifestyle has taken center stage in today's handling of diseases.

A proper diet can tilt you towards living a healthy and enjoyable life as a person. An improper diet would complicate your health, increase suffering and ultimately reduce your quality of life, should it be now or later in the future. You might think about not living a healthy life as digging your own grave. The folly of not living healthy as a person can be compared to pressing a self-destruct button.

Welcome on board! The autophagy flight just took off.

CHAPTER ONE

What is Autophagy?

Did you know the human body is partly cannibalistic by nature?

The body feeds on its unwanted parts. The million-dollar question then is why? Sometimes to achieve our aims or desires we might have to take a step back. Even in construction building, some of the most popular edifices around the world have been adjusted and re-adjusted until the perfect structure was achieved, although in the case of our bodies, consider these adjustments to be constant, as perfection is never really achieved. Autophagy literally means self-eating. It is coined from two words: *auto* (pertaining to self) and *phagy* (eating/devouring).

Autophagy can be defined as the process by which our body reshapes and rebuilds itself, removing unwanted components. It can be defined as the way our body cleans out damaged cells in order to grow new, healthier cells. Autophagy is induced by nutrient limitation and cellular stress, which governs the degradation of the majority of long-lived proteins, protein aggregates and whole organelles. It enables cells to survive stress from both external environment such as nutrient deprivation, as well as internal stress like accumulation of damaged organelles and pathogen invasion.

To put it simply, the body is in search of its masterpiece. Our body pushes itself to the limit, even without our personal effort. It keeps removing unwanted components in a desperate search for non-attainable perfection. On the upside, perfection is very difficult to achieve. Sometimes achieving your own personal best is more than enough.

To highlight the growing effect of autophagy in our world today, the Nobel Assembly at Karolinska Institutet awarded the 2016 Nobel prize in Physiology or Medicine to Yoshinori Ohsumi for his discoveries of the mechanisms of autophagy. Without any doubt, autophagy is not only here to stay, but it is bound to revolutionize medicine altogether.

Basic terminologies

For a better understanding of this book and the brainstorming ideas and principles it embodies, certain terms have to be explained.

Firstly, let's define the term **recycling:** it means to treat or process (used or waste) materials so as to make suitable for reuse: e.g. recycling paper to save trees. Why do we need to recycle? We basically recycle to conserve natural resources, save energy and space. Without recycling there would be heaps of waste everywhere, pollution of the environment and there would be wastage of our limited natural resources.

To recycle means to pass through a series of changes in order to return to a previous stage in a cyclic process. In the context of this book, recycling refers to the way the body degrades cellular components, dead cells, foreign agents, etc. through the aid of lysosomes. Sometimes the degradation process might involve lysing and remodeling. Other times it might just involve lysing, without any remodeling. How does this relate to the human body? For proper functioning, the body must break down damaged or unnecessary organelles and other cellular constituents. Lysosomes are organelles found in the cells of most animal species. They contain digestive enzymes that help to break down biological (related to the body) macro-molecules and foreign bodies. You can call them the soldiers of the autophagic process.

Next is the concept of the **cell:** the cell is the building block of the body. In a building it would be a piece of block, in bread making an ounce of flour and in the constitution it would be the individual clauses, etc. Understanding the cell and its activities is the first step required in understanding autophagy.

The idea behind autophagy

Where did the idea come from? Our bodies where the first scientists to implement autophagy. They have been practicing autophagy long before the first scientists got wind of it. Another good question should be: why does the body deliberately initiate autophagy? Well, the answer to that is a funny one. It has no option. They are stuck with each other.

Even growth is an autophagic process. In growing children and young adults, the body is always shaping and remodeling its tissues to fine-tune the growth process. The scientist is simply trying to understand this amazing technology. Yeah! technology gotten from the body. This should not be surprising, as many ideas behind some of the most groundbreaking discoveries came from natural processes.

Types of autophagy

Cells have two important protein degradation pathways. They are the Ubiquitin Proteasome System (UPS) and the Autophagy-Lysosome Pathway (ALP). The UPS, which is the body's major proteolytic pathway degrades short-lived, soluble proteins while the Autophagy Lysosome Pathway is responsible for degrading or lying older cytoplasmic proteins, soluble and insoluble misfolded proteins, and body organelles. This book is more interested in this second pathway: the **Autophagic Lysosomes Pathway.**

There are three major types of autophagy: **macro-autophagy, micro autophagy and chaperone autophagy**. All three types require certain enzymes and genes to function.

1. Macro-autophagy is one the most important types of autophagy. Its activities are carried out in many parts of the cell. Macro-autophagy is divided in two: the bulk and the selective. Selective macro-autophagy is divided into subtypes. These subtypes are named according to the parts of the cell they target. They are lipophagy (degradation of the lipid part of the cell), pexophagy (degradation of cellular peroxisomes), chlorophagy (degradation of cellular chlorophyll), autophagy (degradation of the mitochondria) and ribophagy (degradation of ribosomes). Other subtypes are emerging, as research on autophagy is still ongoing. In essence, macro-autophagy is concerned with degrading (removing) damaged cell organelles from the cell.

2. Micro-autophagy is more specialized. It involves the direct engulfment of selected materials. This could be foreign bodies such as materials, bacteria, or any element foreign to the body.

3. Chaperone autophagy is the most complex type of autophagy. For chaperone autophagy to take place, a certain protein known as the hsc70 complex must be present. For degradation (lysis) to occur, the particle to be degraded must contain a recognition site for this complex. Binding then occurs at this degradation site (between the recognition site and the hsc70 complex). Chaperone autophagy is the most selective form of autophagy. It screens materials before sending them past the lysosomal barrier.

Why is autophagy activated?

Autophagy is the body's way of responding to stress and physiological conditions. This is an important point to note because it embodies the whole autophagic process, which is the fact that autophagy is always induced. It never occurs on its own, there is always a reason for it. Examples of inducing factors include food deprivation, hyperthermia and hypoxia.

The mechanisms behind autophagy

The autophagic process is a very complex one. However, it was simplified and explained in the most elementary form here. It begins with the formation of a membrane vesicle (usually double stranded). This membrane vesicle then forms a cover around the cell's cytoplasm, altered proteins, old proteins (proteins that have stayed in the cell for a long time) and organelles. It then fuses with autophagic soldiers (lysosomes). The formation of the double-membrane proteins is one of the most important steps in cellular autophagy.

The entire process is regulated by proteins known as "tag proteins". Below are some important autophagic regulators.

Autophagy in steps (autophagic process)

Some of the term descriptions are pretty advanced. However, understanding them would help you grasp autophagy better. The terms were simplified as much as possible.

1. Sequestration

This is the first step in the autophagy process. During this stage, two membranes expand and cover the cytoplasm. These membranes are known as phagophores. The phagophore does not only enclose the cytoplasm. It equally encloses the organelles within it. The purpose of enclosing them (cytoplasm and organelles) is to prepare them for degradation. Before the end of this stage, the phagophore becomes an organelle called the autophagosome.

2. Transportation

Earlier in the book when we discussed terminologies, we described lysosomes as autophagic soldiers. That rank was well deserved, as the whole autophagic process revolves around them. For degradation to occur, the autophagosome has to connect with the lysosome. Essentially, the transportation stage (step 2) involves the formation of structures that will aid the transfer of materials from the autophagosome to the lysosome.

In order to connect with the lysosomes, the autophagosome fuses with an intermediate organelle called the endosome. Together, they form what is called an amphisome. The amphisome can readily fuse with the lysosomes.

3. Lysing/degradation

This is the final step in the autophagy process. The amphisome fuses with the lysosome, conveying its contents. The lysosome then releases enzymes known as hydrolases. They lyse (degrade) all the materials conveyed from the amphisome. The resulting structure, which now consists of degraded cellular material, is now called an autolysosome. The degraded products (amino acids) are now transported from the autolysosome into the cellular fluid. They are either marked for excretion or can be used to build new cells.

Autophagic regulators

-Insulin/IGF-1

Although Atg proteins are the major regulators in the autophagic process, the insulin/IGF-1 pathway plays a vital role. The pathway promotes growth, morphogenesis and survival.

Nutrient deprivation also plays a role in autophagy. The body tries to generate nutrients for itself. It does this by lysing (degrading) old and worn out cells and using them as a nutrient source. To carry this out, an Atg protein is hyper-phosphorylated by TORC1.

Apart from its role in nutrient generation (autophagic pathway), TORC1 equally contributes to the activation of several factors that oversee transcription or translation of some proteins by phosphorylation. Some of these proteins are needed (utilized) in the autophagic pathway. TOR regulates the induction of autophagy. It does this alongside protein kinase A and SCh9.

-DRAM and p53

The p53 suppressor is found in about half of the human population. It exists in a mutated form and helps to induce autophagy. It is equally important in helping the body to carry out apoptosis. Apoptosis simply means programmed cell death.

-FOXO and ROS

Recent research has shown that FOXO aids in the transcription of autophagy related genes. Some of these genes include Atg8/LC3, Atg12, Vps34, and Atg6. In muscles undergoing atrophy, Atg6 induces protein degradation in the atrophied cells.

ROS (Reactive Oxygen Species) have been found to play a role in starvation induced autophagy. During starvation, the body degrades (breaks down) old cells. Some of the nutrients from these degraded cells are then moved to more important cells. You can compare this to a generator powering a whole building. In a situation where the fuel tank has very little fuel left in it, a compromise has to be reached. The generator operator would have to reduce the load.

Unimportant devices are turned off, while the important devices are kept running.

CHAPTER TWO:
How To Achieve Autophagy

Boosting autophagy in your body simply means trying to make your body operate at its optimum. You are maximizing your output and increasing your body's efficiency. Amazingly, not only is your body operating at its maximum, but it is operating on **clean energy.** You can call this the body's version of green energy. You are supplying your body with nutrients and energy in the cleanest (healthiest) way possible.

There are three major ways to boost autophagy in the body.

Keto diet

This is a simple and natural way of activating autophagy without forgoing some of your favorite meals. The idea is to reduce carbohydrate levels. When carbohydrate levels are low, the body has no choice but to use fat as a fuel source. This is the concept behind the extremely popular ketogenic diet.

Keto diets are diets high in fat and low in carbohydrates (e.g. teak, bacon and peanut butter shakes). Between 60 and 70 percent of your overall calories come from fat. Proteins are the next major contributors. They make up about 20 to 30% of the body's calories.

Protein provides 20 to 30 percent of calories, while only 5 percent comes from carbs. This shows that carbohydrates are the most insignificant part of our diet. While proteins can be converted into sugar (in the absence of carbohydrates), fats cannot.

So basically, in ketosis you lose excess body fat while retaining muscle. Ketogenesis equally aids the body in resolving cancerous tumors, lowers the risk of diabetes and protects the body from brain disorders such as epilepsy. Ketosis can be said to be an autophagy hack. Through keto-diets you can gain the benefits of autophagy, without stressing your body too much. In keto-diets there is a gradual shift from burning carbs (glucose) to ketones. Autophagy is keto-based, hence very little carb is involved in autophagy.

Fasting

-Water Fasting

Water fasting is a milder form of fasting. Fasting (in all forms) is one of the most effective ways of achieving autophagy. An individual undergoing a water fast can drink water. Although he or she will not consume anything else except water for twenty-four hours, water fasts might not be as effective as a full fast. A full fast does not involve water. Nothing is eaten within twenty-four hours. Water fasting benefits include weight loss, body cleansing, cellular regeneration and, most importantly, autophagy. It is increasing in popularity.

Also, the presence of oxygen in the water helps the body. It assists the body in eliminating harmful toxins. That is why water fasting is nicknamed the expert cleanser. Whenever water and fasting meet, detoxification must occur.

Water is calorie-free. That is why water enhances metabolism and ketogenesis. There are links between drinking water and weight loss. As the body shifts to ketosis during water fasting, it can use up excess fat. Water fasting also boosts the body's healing process. It reduces inflammation in the body and lowers blood sugar levels while enhancing the activities of the heart and brain. Additionally, drinking water supports collagen synthesis in the skin.

Tips (on water fasting)

Fasting requires a lot of effort. Before you begin a water fast, you need to prepare yourself mentally. You need to always picture the light at the end of the tunnel. Visualizing your goals will help motivate you.

Before commencing your water fast, you should have a doctor's consultation to decide the duration of your program.

Abstaining from food for a week and taking nothing but water can be very tough especially at the beginning. You might feel hungry or weak as your body will be in a state of ketosis after 3-4 days. The body adapts to this 'new' system and the fasting process becomes much easier.

Setting the duration of your fast

Fasting essentially means abstinence from all foods. In Islam or Christianity for example, fasting dates are based for days of the week, months or a year. It can be done for different durations.

Water fasting can last for as little as 3 days to a whole month based on the objective and capability of the person. For example, it is suggested that individuals suffering from chronic illnesses should avoid water fasts longer than 3 days.

The amount of water taken in a day is directly related to the individual's level of activity. Although the amount of water taken in is not critical (in respect to results), most people, irrespective of the amount of water they drink, experience tremendous changes (weight loss, detoxification, autophagy, etc.).

-Skipping meals/intermittent fasting

Skipping meals is another method you can use to achieve autophagy. Unlike ketosis, this method is stressful. At first you might not understand the benefits, but you are bound to become addicted once you start seeing the results. Recent studies have shown that periodic fasting and autophagy can make cancer treatments more productive. Normal body cells are not affected unlike in normal cancer therapy. Modern cancer therapies are very harsh. They make wholesale changes to your body size (weight) and can even affect your looks.

Recent research has shown that intermittent fasting improves brain function, brain structure and neuroplasticity. It helps the brain to reorganize and replenish itself. It equally helps to improve cognitive function and structures.

Intermittent fasting is simply taking skipping meals to another level. Intermittent fasting should be adopted to suit your capabilities and personal targets. Whichever way you choose to practice it, you are bound to reap some amazing benefits. Some of these benefits include increased resistance to diseases and infection, reduced body weight, increased lifespan, improved cardiovascular function, increased brain function and a whole lot more.

Children, pregnant women, people with ulcers, low sugar levels and persons with food associated ailments (diseases) are advised to practice intermittent fasting mildly. In some cases, they should avoid it totally, most especially pregnant women.

So then, the question is: *How can intermittent fasting improve autophagy?* Well let's compare this to a packed fridge. This fridge belongs to Mr. Food (hypothetic). He keeps packing his fridge with food. The fridge is now in layers (layers of food). Some of these foods reach their expiry dates. Mr. Food can't see or notice this. Naturally, decomposition begins, followed by a foul odor. Cool story, right?

This mirrors what happens in our bodies when we keep over feeding. The body is packed up with digestion products (glucose, fat, amino acids) that keep piling up. There's a popular adage: "**too much of anything is never good".** This is a universal truth. Our bodies, the atmosphere, water, soil, etc., all exist on a delicate balance. Nature finds a way to balance itself. No excesses, just perfection!

Intermittent fasting is one of the ways we can help our body to achieve this balance. Fasting forces the body to use up its stores. Some cells die during this process (autophagy). These cells are replaced by the body when you feed again. *Hence, the body is renewed and refreshed!*

-Longer fasts (no food or water)

Intermittent fasting is a vital tool for improving health, achieving weight loss, detoxification, cellular regeneration and autophagy. There is enough evidence to back this up. However, longer fasts have proven to be more effective. *Please, always fast according to your capabilities. You can achieve similar results with both water fasts, intermittent fasts and full fasts.*

Full fasting can take many forms. The most drastic is a "dry fast", which entails avoiding all edibles and fluids (food or water). **Never start a full fast without consulting a medical practitioner.** Full fasts can be very severe and shouldn't be done for more than 48 hours.

Long fasts and autophagy

The most outstanding benefit of full fasts is their ability to induce autophagy. If you abstain from food, your body will be forced to use up its stores. Old cells are recycled as well. They are used to build new cells (autophagy). After 24 hours, the body uses up most of the glycogen in the liver.

In respect to weight loss, the body loses around 1-2 pounds a day. This happens because it is shedding water weight and protein. However, the body's dependence on protein as a source of energy is short-lived. Using protein would mean breaking down muscles, some of which might be essential/delicate.

This makes fat a more reliable/suitable energy source. Hence, after a few days, the body switches to its fat stores for energy (ketosis). Fat is more energy-dense per pound than protein, so weight loss in this phase is slower. It reduces to just over 1 pound every 2 days.

A long fast is the easiest way of staying in ketosis for an extended duration. It forces the body to rely completely on its own fat stores instead of dietary fat. Being in ketosis makes weight loss easy. Ketosis helps suppress hunger (especially after the first few days, which are usually tough). Fasting also enables you to totally get your mind off food. It saves you the stress of thinking about what to eat next and bothering on the amount of food you are eating.

Full fast is an effective means to lose a lot of weight quickly. However, many people begin to gain it all back again because they just go back to their old eating pattern.

Like most "crash diets," fasting will help you lose weight, but won't help you maintain the status quo, unless you also make permanent changes in your diet after the fast is over.

As we noted earlier, long fasts promote autophagy, which can be compared to "spring cleaning" for your cells. Since the body is basically eating itself, it has a chance to eliminate any junk or waste products that may have built up, and repair the harm caused by oxidative stress. This is one of the substantial benefits of fasting even for people who have a healthy weight. Autophagy also has powerful anti-aging and muscle-building properties.

Recent research has shown that an extended fast (10 days on average) was beneficial to people suffering from hypertension, also noting that even though the patients didn't start the fasting program to lose weight, all of them had an average weight loss of around 15 pounds. Full fasts (up to 5 days) may also have some benefits for chemotherapy patients.

Another effect of full fasts is mental clarity. It is a way to break free from overeating patterns or other food disorders. Fasting is practiced by many religious groups because it enhances meditation and mindfulness. Briefly put, fasting declogs the mind and increases focus.

Exercise

Working out stresses the muscles (damages them in a good way). The muscles are torn and rebuilt. This makes them stronger and more resistant. Increasing your muscular strength improves your body's condition. People who exercise regularly are less prone to diseases and infections. Researchers have discovered that exercise improves the human immune system. Resistance training is usually the most effective type of exercise, not just for autophagy, but the body as a whole. When done at intervals, the body's conditioning improves. You tear up your muscles, rebuild stronger ones and stimulate autophagy.

Exercise is in essence a physical method of achieving autophagy. You use up your body stores directly when you exercise. Most people describe exercise as refreshing. Well, that is not just a feeling. It is actually happening. *Exercise catalyzes regeneration* (development of new cells). To regenerate means to replace lost or damaged tissue. So not only are new cells being produced, old ones are encouraged to die.

Exercising is very important in the treatment of any disease. How rigorous the exercise is, depends on your doctor's approval. Exercise improves your body's use of insulin and may lower blood sugar levels apart from helping to use up some of the excess glucose. Exercise equally helps to increase blood circulation, enhance kidney function, reduce risk of developing diabetes and in general helps to improve the body's condition.

Exercise can equally lower the chance of having a heart attack or stroke and can improve circulation. Furthermore, it has been proven that exercise benefits the brain greatly. It increases blood circulation to the brain and helps increase the brain's efficiency. Exercise is highly recommended, especially for those who are obese/overweight. Care should be taken not to over work the body in one go. Exercise should be gradual and progressive. A minimum of 150 minutes a week (total exercise time) is recommended.

A large number of diseases target and attack the muscles. They reduce their mass, finally rendering them useless. The body cannot function without strong muscles. Exercising daily helps your body keep its muscles alive and strong.

You do not have to follow a drastic, severe exercising program. All you have to do is try to exercise at least three hours a week. Walking in a park for an hour, running on a treadmill, going to the mall for three hours, in other words simply walking around often is a good start to keep your body in shape. When you go shopping, try to park far from the entrance so you have to walk more on your way there and back.

Exercising helps your blood circulate through your body and helps your body burn fat and bad calories. By exercising, the sugar in your blood is used to help your muscles function and therefore not be stagnant in your organs and arteries. It is a simple process: more you eat, more you need to exercise and more you exercise, more you need to eat.

According to doctors and researchers, exercising is the best way to fight disease. However, it does so with a daily routine or at least a tri-weekly habit. Just walking around the block once a month is not enough, extra effort is needed.

Exercising helps you feel better about yourself as it releases endorphins in your body, the same endorphins you would get by eating your favorite food. Working out fights the high level of cholesterol and keeps cholesterol related diseases away.

If you plan on exercising daily and at a high level, talk about it with your doctor. He will help you find the best program for your needs and physical and medical abilities. You will have to take it slowly, step by step. Do not try to run a marathon on the first day or go on a five-mile run because you want to burn the calories. You will burn as many calories walking a mile at a good pace as you would by running the same distance.

Dietary tips

To achieve autophagy, you can try some of these dietary tips. At least once or twice a week, you should limit your protein intake to 15-25 grams a day. This gives the body nearly a day to recycle stored proteins, reduce inflammation and cleanse body cells. The best part is that the muscle mass remains the same. It does not shrink or reduce. During this abstinence period (food abstinence), the body is forced to consume its stored proteins and toxins. Skipping breakfast (say twice a week), helps to promote autophagy in the body. It gives the body time to clean itself (eliminate lingering toxins).

Research has shown that about 30% of women respond to intermittent fasting more severely. To curb these effects, a fat-based breakfast is recommended. Basically, you are required to keep carbohydrates and fat from your meals (for a whole day). However, the quantity taken should be regulated. Fats are energy Kings. Half of kilogram of fat gives three or four times more energy than proteins or carbohydrates of the same quantity. So, taking in a very small quantity of fat is usually more than enough. This way, you are not starving your body, while promoting autophagy.

Your daily meals have a direct effect on your body. Some foods, when consumed in large quantities are unhealthy, while others have minimal or no negative effects on the body. Therefore, managing what you eat, knowing the calorie content, the ingredients and how they affect your body is very important. Generally, three major classes of food appear in most of our meals or diets. They include carbohydrates, fats and proteins. Vegetables, fruits and fiber appear much less in meals and diets. To influence your health positively, an understanding of these food classes and their effects on the body is very important.

Carbohydrates

These are one of the most popular food classes. They exist as starches, sugar and fiber in foods such as grains, fruits, vegetables, milk products and sweets. They increase blood sugar levels and affect the body more than any other food. Therefore, knowing what foods contain carbohydrates and regulating the amount per meal is helpful for blood glucose control. Carbohydrates in your meal should come from healthy sources like vegetables, fruits, whole grains and legumes. Also, carbohydrates coming from whole grain (high fibers) are recommended. Those originating from sources with added sugars, fats and salt should be avoided.

Carbohydrate control and regulation is the bedrock to achieving autophagy. Eating carbohydrates is not bad (unhealthy) in essence. The quantity simply has to be reduced, and carbohydrates from healthier sources should be integrated into meal plans. Eating carbohydrates from healthy sources can equally help you to lose excess body weight and generally make you healthier.

Proteins

Proteins are an important part of our diet. In an experiment where an individual consumed a given quantity of protein and another consumed the same quantity of carbohydrates, the individual who took the carbohydrates was most likely to be hungry first. This shows how important proteins are in helping create satiety. Proteins mildly contribute to the glucose (sugar levels) in the body and are usually increased in most recommended meal plans (health meal plans). However, to achieve autophagy, proteins are not needed in high quantities. Proteins are equally the building blocks of the body, and generally help the body to recover from stress and ailments.

Fats

These are the number one energy givers in the body. Fats are an important component in the creation of balanced diets, and more importantly, in achieving autophagy. When digested, fats undergo ketosis (an important energy cycle the body experiences in times of starvation). Therefore, when you take the right amount of fats, you can induce artificial starvation. Most especially healthy fats are from fish (e.g. trout and salmon), nuts, seeds, olive oil, canola oil, other vegetable oils, avocado, and soft margarine. Fats don't raise blood glucose but are high in calories. Their high calorie content and energy giving ability means that very small quantities can sustain the body. Health wise, it is advisable to use non-saturated fatty acids as against saturated fatty acids. Sources of saturated fatty acids include butter, red meat, cakes, pastries and deep-fried foods. Instead, plant-based protein and lower fat dairy products should be used more often.

Generally, to create an autophagy inducing diet, fats should be included more in the diet, albeit in differing quantities.

Vegetables and fruit

Vegetables and fruits are beneficial to the body. They help in flushing and cleansing the body. They contain many vitamins and minerals to help supply vital nutrients and regulate vital body activities. They can equally be used as snacks, because most of them contain fibers. Hence, they can easily cause satiety. Fruits also contain natural sugars which are less harmful to the body.

Other methods to induce autophagy

-Drugs

Although the use of drugs to achieve autophagy is still relatively untested (in its infancy), certain drugs have the ability to induce autophagy. Although their actions are usually specific (inducing their effects in certain parts of the body), their actions are not generalized.

For example, latrepirdine, resveratrol and lithium are used to stimulate autophagy in patients with Huntington's disease. Since research is presently ongoing, their usage is still very limited.

In the treatment of Alzheimer's disease, certain drugs/substances such as nicotinamide, hydroxy chloroquine, resveratrol, nilotinib, lithium, latrepirdine, metformin, valproic acid and statins have been credited with inducing different levels of autophagy. Equally, in the treatment of Parkinson's disease nilotinib and statins have been credited with inducing autophagy. Lastly, lithium, tamoxifen, and valproic are said to be capable of inducing Amyotrophic lateral sclerosis (ALS).

Most of these drugs are relatively untested. However, advancements are being made as we speak. Their usage is currently limited to neurodegenerative and auto-immune diseases. In the future, it is hoped that autophagy would be more widely used.

-Regulating sleep

It is recommended that we get at least 7-9 hours of sleep a day. Despite these recommendations, modern research has shown that the amount of sleep an individual requires depends on his or her sleep personality. This factor is scientifically called the sleep chronotype. Studies have shown that about 4 sleep personalities exist. Each sleep personality requires a certain amount of sleep a day (different sleep combinations). Certain individuals (based on their sleep personality) can cope with less sleep, while others require more. Sleep plays an important role in body recovery (regeneration of cells). Therefore, knowing the exact amount of sleep you need per day is very important. However, it should be noted that sleep is qualitative and not quantitative. Sleeping for hours under duress and in uncomfortable conditions might not be beneficial for the body.

Less hours of sleep in a comfortable and relaxed environment, position or place might be worth more.

-Drink coffee

Modern research has shown that caffeine can induce autophagy in the muscle tissue, liver and heart. Even when taken on a full stomach or with other foods, its ability to induce autophagy is not reduced.

-Turmeric

Turmeric has proven to be effective in inducing autophagy in the cell, specifically in the mitochondria. This is majorly due to curcumin, a nutrient found in turmeric.

-Virgin olive oil

Virgin olive oil contains an antioxidant called oleuropein. Oleuropein is said to have anti-cancerous properties, one of which stems from its ability to induce autophagy.

-Ginger

Ginger consumption can help induce autophagy. This is because ginger contains an active component called 6-shogaol. 6-shogaol has become renowned for its efficiency in the treatment of lung cancer.

-Green Tea

The ingredient responsible for the autophagic ability of green tea is called polyphenol. It is found in both green and white tea. It is organ-specific, with most of its actions focused on the liver, where it helps to prevent inflammation, cancer and liver damage.

-Coconut Oil

Coconut oil is rich in ketones. Ketones are natural components produced by the body in times of starvation. Hence, by taking coconut oil, you are inducing starvation (a fake one) in the body.

-Reishi Mushroom

Even before its autophagy inducing properties where discovered, Reishi mushrooms where used in traditional medicine for decades in Asia. Modern research has shown that Reishi mushrooms can induce autophagy, which in turn produces anticancer effects in those who suffer from breast cancer.

-Vitamin D

Also known as the sunshine vitamin, vitamin D is synthesized naturally in the body (specifically in the skin). Its precursors are activated by sunlight. Those staying in regions where sunlight is minimal or non-existent (e.g. artic regions) might have to take synthesized vitamin D.

Vitamin D is capable of inducing autophagy in the pancreatic islets. Predictably, this will increase insulin production in the pancreas and is therefore very effective in the treatment of type 2 diabetes.

-Melatonin

Melatonin is the only hormone on this list. It plays an important role in the regulation of our circadian rhythm (circadian rhythm is very important in coordinating sleep). Recent studies have shown that melatonin supplementation can induce autophagy in the brain. It helps to protect the brain from cell injury. Cellular injury is one of the leading causes of neuropsychiatric conditions around the world.

-Ginseng (ginseng root)

Ginseng is one of the most important natural supplements in the world today. It is sold around the globe and is even capable of boosting the human immune system. Apart from its immune boosting ability, it also induces autophagy and helps prevent cancer.

CHAPTER THREE

Autophagy in weight loss

Autophagy benefits the body, whether you are overweight or not. However, we will first analyze its use in the treatment of excess body weight.

Excess body weight has been associated with the development of many diseases in the world today. If finding the cause of diseases (a random pick) was tried in a court of law, excess body weight would be incriminated, probably with countless charges. The role it plays in the development of diseases cannot be overstated.

For starters, when is a person said to be overweight? An overweight person is described as heavier than what is generally considered healthy for a given body type and height. Most people don't even know if they are overweight.

How to know if you are overweight:

If in advanced cases an obese individual can easily be assessed visually, this might prove to be difficult in individuals who are only slightly overweight or obese. There are two recommended methods to check this: by referring to the body mass index method and by measuring the waste size.

-Body Mass Index Method

This method measures the weight of a person in relation to his or her height. A score is obtained from the calculation, which is then used to categorize the individual. Normal weight individuals usually fall into a body mass index of about 18.5 to 24.9, while overweight individuals usually fall into a body mass index of about 25.0 and above.

-Waist size

This is another method used in checking the body weight statistics of a person. Overall, having too much fat around the waistline is very unhealthy.

For women, having a waist size of more than 35 inches is seen as unhealthy while for men anything more than a waist size of 40 is seen as inappropriate.

Autophagy and excess body weight

What's the secret behind losing weight? Some would say exercise, others might say dieting, while others still might recommend a product (slimming teas, fat burning creams, etc.). The truth is that you cannot lose weight effectively without discipline, which is why stimulating autophagy is the best way to lose weight. Why is this? Because autophagy is the definition of discipline (in terms of health). Autophagy is a combination of dieting, exercising and every other healthy way of losing fat.

There is no need to sugar-coat things. If you do not have a reasonable amount of self-discipline, you might never achieve autophagy effectively.

How it works

Autophagy simply means cell eating. This definition is shorter than the one given in the beginning of the book but is nevertheless a good one.

Autophagy cleans up the body. We previously told a short fictional story about Mr. Food. He packed his fridge with food, some of which was perishable. Even when the fridge got full, he kept adding. The fridge was full to the brim. Some of the items started decomposing, and as expected, the fridge developed a bad smell. Mr. Food didn't stop though. He kept adding more and more food because he loved it too much to let go.

This story might sound funny or ridiculous, but it really describes the way most people treat their body. They keep on packing it with unwanted materials (food). You gain weight when your body builds its muscles. However, when food is in excess, especially for people who live a sedentary type of life, the body begins to deposit these excesses in body tissues, organs and the muscles.

The result is an increase in weight (overweight/obese).

Autophagy excels when the body is put to stress. The word stress should not scare you. It just involves living a disciplined and healthy life. You can achieve weight loss through autophagy by following the steps listed in 'how to achieve autophagy'.

And in normal individuals?

It would be a huge mistake to exclude yourself from the recommended steps because you are not overweight. The body always has excesses to burn.

Autophagy in Metabolic Diseases

To a large extent, autophagy borders on what we eat. It is therefore not surprising that it plays a huge role in the body's defense against metabolic diseases.

Metabolic diseases are those diseases that are affected or related to the body's digestion of food. Diabetes is the most popular metabolic disease. *Advancements in autophagy research has been giving more insight into treatment of the disease.*

To understand the role autophagy plays in modern treatment of diabetes, we would have to first understand diabetes (analyze the disease).

Before we move on to how autophagy aids in the treatment of diabetes, we will take a brief look at the symptoms of the disease. Symptom detection has become very important in our world today. *Early detection of any symptom could be the sharp line between life and death.* Nowadays, diabetes is one of the most widespread diseases in the world.

Diagnosis of any medical condition is usually achieved in two ways. One is by observing the characteristic symptoms of the disease. That is to say every disease has its characteristic symptoms or conditions. The second way is through clinical diagnosis. This involves carrying out certain tests on the selected individual.

Diagnosis Using Symptoms

Type 1 and type 2 diabetes share common symptoms. First among them is:

-Weakness/Tiredness/Hunger

Diabetes messes up with the body's energy metabolism. When insulin is not produced in the required quantity, glucose is not properly transported to the body's organs, cells and muscles. *Autophagy reduces this dependence on glucose. An autophagy diet supplies the body with essential nutrients and energy.*

Earlier in the book, we stated how important nutrients are to the body. Diabetes patients will experience weakness due to lack of energy. This weakness is due to an imbalance in the body's energy mechanism. *Autophagy helps correct this!* Tiredness and hunger can equally result from lack of or reduced energy in a diabetic.

-Frequent Urination and Increased Thirst

Like every symptom of diabetes, these symptoms are also linked to glucose metabolism (breakdown). In this case, excess glucose is transported to the kidney as a result of glucose under-utilization. The kidney would normally absorb some of this glucose, but in this case the quantity to be absorbed makes it impossible. Hence, the kidney transports (sends) a part of the excess glucose (that could not be absorbed) into the urine. This process occurs quite often, which causes the frequent urination.

Autophagy reduces the body's dependence on glucose. It creates healthier energy pathways, which prevent all that was listed above. The kidneys have less glucose to process/absorb, consequently reducing the quantity of urine released.

Like all bodily fluids, urine contains water. As a result, frequent urination will lead to dehydration, which is signaled by its own specific symptoms. Thirst is one of the most frequent symptoms that occur in diabetes. And like always, one thing leads to another. Thirst would cause the affected individual to drink more water. In return, drinking more water will lead to increased urine output (frequent urination). Other symptoms such as dryness of the skin, dizziness and tiredness might be experienced as well.

-Dehydration Symptoms

As explained earlier, dehydration is a condition that results from frequent urination caused by diabetes. In more severe cases, other symptoms of dehydration will become more pronounced. These include dizziness, dryness of the skin, itchy skin, dryness of the mouth, blurred vision (result of the changing fluids in the eyes, specifically the retina) and many more.

-Yeast Infections

People suffering from type 2 diabetes are prone to yeast infections. Glucose (sugar) is a natural substrate for yeast. Therefore, the overabundance of glucose that occurs in diabetes promotes the growth of yeast, and invariably yeast infections. (*Autophagy helps to reduce the body's dependence on glucose - reduced blood sugar levels*). Yeast infections are known to grow in the moist parts of the body. This includes between the fingers and sometimes around the pubic region area and under the breasts.

-Difficulty for Wounds to Heal

High blood sugar levels affect the blood's ability to clot and coagulate (hinders the blood clotting pathway).

-Sharp Loss in Weight

Following damage to the pancreas and the resulting reduction in body glucose levels, the body has to find an alternative source of energy to carry out its numerous activities. It turns to its fatty stores (muscles around the body) and breaks them down, thus creating a new pathway for energy. Continuous breakdown in body fat leads to loss of weight. This process occurs quite quickly which brings about the sharp loss in weight. *Autophagy ensures the body's fatty stores are replenished. It balances the body's energy mechanism and increases overall efficiency.*

Classical Symptoms of Gestational Diabetes

The symptoms occurring in gestational diabetes are not exclusive to it. They also include normal diabetes symptoms such as thirst, frequent urination, tiredness/weakness and sometimes loss of weight.

The metabolic syndrome and CHD

The first abnormality in type 2 diabetes is insulin resistance. It is found in people even before diabetes can be diagnosed. It simply means that your body becomes resistant to the effects of insulin and finds it increasingly difficult over time to keep your blood sugar down to a normal level. When insulin resistance is found in combination with other risk factors, it is called metabolic syndrome (the same combination used to be known as insulin resistance syndrome). About 1 in 4 adults in the UK has metabolic syndrome, and while not all of them have diabetes now, many or even most of them will go on to develop it unless they do some serious work to improve their lifestyle (adopting healthier and more productive living patterns - Autophagic lifestyle).

The International Diabetes Federation has come up with a definition of the metabolic syndrome that involves having at least three of the risk factors listed in the book. Each of them on their own increases the risk of CHD. Add them together, and they more than triple your risk of CHD compared to someone who doesn't have them.

Diabetes and autophagy

Autophagy plays an important role in regulating the activities of the pancreatic islets. It helps to stimulate insulin secretion, especially in times of crisis (low insulin levels). Insulin helps to balance glucose levels in the body.

Not only does autophagy stimulate insulin secretion, it equally helps to protects the pancreatic islets from oxidative stress. In-vitro and in-vivo studies (inside and outside the body) have also shown that autophagy plays a role in their function and survival (pancreatic islets).

Autophagy counters the destructive effects of apoptosis. Apoptosis means programmed cell death. Just like autophagy, apoptosis is a naturally occurring process in the body. However, apoptosis can be mis-controlled, leading to the destruction of body cells that where not marked for destruction.

CHAPTER FOUR: Autophagy in Neurodegenerative Disorders

Medical and scientific research has shown that *neuronal autophagy* plays a critical role in maintaining the body's cellular activities. It plays an equally important role in maintaining nervous system health. Autophagy clears up aggregated proteins. Many scientists believe that these aggregated proteins are behind the development of many neurodegenerative diseases.

In past times, it was believed that neuronal autophagy had little or no effects on the development of neurodegenerative diseases. However, recent studies have revealed the importance of autophagy in non-proliferating cells, particularly in body neurons.

Autophagy plays a vital role in neuroprotection, by implementing multiple key molecular regulations of autophagy pathway.

Autophagy helps revive the body's cells, especially those under stress. Autophagy equally aids in the maintenance of cellular homeostasis. Increasing evidence indicates that autophagy machineries are derailed in diverse human diseases, including most neurodegenerative disorders, cancers and inflammatory disorders. Derailed autophagy contributes to neuron degeneration and neuronal cell death disease pathology.

Plenty of evidence has shown the importance of autophagy in the regulation of neurodegenerative disorders. A better understanding of neuronal autophagy will ultimately help medical practitioners develop potential therapeutic interventions targeting autophagic dysregulation.

A part of these neurodegenerative disorders will be discussed below, along with the contributions of autophagy to their treatment.

Parkinson's disease

This is a neurodegenerative disease. Autophagy plays a huge role in the regulation of these diseases. Parkinson's disease is a progressive nervous system disease that affects movement. Symptoms have a slow onset, usually with a barely noticeable tremor in one part of the body, generally the hands. Although tremors are the most popular symptom, other symptoms such as stiffness or slowing of movement might be found.

In the initial stages of Parkinson's disease, the face becomes nearly expressionless. Arms become stiff and movement becomes almost robotic. Speech becomes incoherent and unclear. The disease worsens with time.

Currently, Parkinson's disease is incurable, and medications are palliative. In more complex forms of the disease, surgery might be required to reduce its effects.

Symptoms

As previously stated, any discussion on a disease without proper analysis of the symptoms is incomplete. Early detection of a disease's symptoms would most likely make treatment more effective.

Signs and symptoms of Parkinson's disease are not consistent. Early (mild) signs usually go unnoticed. Most of the time, symptoms begin on one side of the body, and they usually remain worse on that side as the condition progresses

Frequently encountered symptoms:

-Tremor

Tremors usually begin in the extremities. The most popular is rubbing of the thumb and forefinger back-and-forth. This is known as a pill-rolling tremor. Tremors might continue even when the body is at rest. Parkinson's disease slows down movements, making easy actions look very complex. Movement becomes restricted, and some patients might need assistance or a walking stick.

-Rigid muscles

Muscles become very rigid and stiff.

-Impaired posture and balance

Posture becomes irregular, patients appear to bend, walk irregularly or without balance.

-Poor reflexes

Reflex actions become more difficult. Patients can even find it difficult to blink.

-Speech changes

Patients' tone of voice becomes soft and irregular. Sometimes the voice might be altered completely.

-Difficulty in writing

Writing becomes very difficult or nearly impossible.

-Presence of Lewy bodies

This symptom can't be seen with the naked eye. It requires a clinical test, after which it is analyzed by medical personnel.

Lewy bodies are important in the diagnosis of Parkinson's disease, and their appearance is almost confirmatory of the presence of the disease.

If you have any of the above symptoms, seek medical advice/assistance.

Causes

Parkinson's disease results from the destruction of the brain's nerve cells. Almost all symptoms have nervous links or origins. Attack on the nerve cells usually affects dopamine levels (dopamine is a neurotransmitter associated with the feeling of pleasure). It is usually this decrease in dopamine levels that causes the symptoms.

Parkinson's disease is currently incurable! We will soon discuss the role autophagy plays in its treatment.

Parkinson's disease and autophagy

Researchers believe that regular exercise (anaerobic exercise) and caffeine consumption can help reduce chances of developing the disease. It is not surprising that both of them promote autophagy.

Some of the pathologies associated with Parkinson's disease (PD) are oxidative stress, mitochondrial dysfunction and protein aggregation. They are all linked with autophagy. Autophagy had previously been regarded as a nutrient based body response. However, increasing recent research has shown that basal and constitutive autophagy is needed for neuronal survival and that its in-availability can lead to neurodegeneration.

Recent research has demonstrated that alteration in autophagic pathway can result in the formation of abnormal proteins. This is commonly observed in neurodegenerative diseases, such as Alzheimer's, Huntington's and Parkinson's diseases. In addition, many of the proteins related to Parkinson's disease, such as PINK1 and PARKIN, have an important role in the process of autophagy. Autophagy is part of the cell's self-maintenance machinery. Thus, maintaining a proper level of autophagy is important for reducing abnormal protein aggregates.

Discovery of drugs/substances that can boost autophagic activity could significantly reduce neuronal loss, preventing the progression of the disease. A clearer understanding of the regulatory processes involved in autophagic pathogenesis of PD will facilitate the identification of feasible methods for clinical application.

Alzheimer's disease

Alzheimer's disease is a progressive neurodegenerative disorder that causes brain cells and tissues to degenerate. Alzheimer's disease is the number one cause of dementia. It influences thinking, behavioral and social skills making the affected person to appear confused.

Affected individuals have a tendency to forget recent events and conversations. In later stages, patients suffering from Alzheimer's disease will develop severe memory impairment (sometimes permanent impairment) and might find it difficult to perform everyday tasks.

Treatment might temporarily improve symptoms or reduce the rate of decline. These treatments are very useful for patients suffering from Alzheimer's disease as they can help them improve the quality of their life, helping them maintain independence for some time. Modern programs and services have been created to help support patients with Alzheimer's disease and their caregivers.

Like many other neurodegenerative diseases, Alzheimer's disease is not curable at the present time. Alzheimer's disease alters brain function and can cause in advanced stages severe complications such as loss of brain function, dehydration, malnutrition, infection and even death.

Symptoms

Memory loss is the predominant symptom of Alzheimer's disease. The first symptom of the disease is usually difficulty to remember recent events and conversations. Total or partial memory loss might result later.

At first, people with Alzheimer's disease may be aware of their shortcomings (newfound forgetfulness).

Brain alterations associated with Alzheimer's disease lead to growing trouble with memory. We all have occasional lapses in memory. It's normal to lose track of one or two things from time to time. The memory loss associated with Alzheimer's disease is different. It often persists and worsens with time, affecting a person's ability to carry out tasks independently.

Individuals suffering from Alzheimer's disease would routinely exhibit the following:

-Forget discussions/conversations, forget events and even names of family members (children, spouses, siblings) or even forget them totally.

-Casually misplace possessions, usually putting them in obscure places.

-Usually make poor conversations. They might find it difficult to make out sentences or reason out words. They always seem to be in a world of their own.

In relation to their thoughts and reasoning, they might exhibit the following:

-Might find it difficult to concentrate on a particular thing.

-Multitasking becomes nearly impossible. Patients usually forget important things. Alzheimer patients should not be left on their own. There should always be someone around them.

-The ability to make rational decisions and judgments declines gradually. Patients might make unusual or uncharacteristic choices such as social interactions and choice of clothing.

-Might find it difficult to perform routine tasks or activities like cooking, playing games and even grooming (dressing and bathing).

Patients might have changes in behavior or character. Patients might exhibit the following:

-Seasonal depression,

-Social withdrawal,

-Frequent mood swings,

-Becoming very suspicious (develop theories),

-Increased aggression,

-Unusual sleeping patterns,

-Wandering about or getting lost,

-Unpredictability.

Memorized skills

Memorized skills are kept for longer periods of time, even in the latter stages of the disease. Memorized skills may include studying, defense, storytelling, singing, listening to music, dancing, drawing and sculpting.

Researchers say these skills are preserved longer because they are governed by paths of the brain that only become affected when the disease worsens.

If you experience any of these symptoms, consider seeing a doctor.

Causes

There is no designated cause. However, scientists think the disease results from a combination of genetic, lifestyle and environmental factors that alter the brain's normal functioning.

A meager one percent of Alzheimer's cases is caused by genetic alterations. Individuals that display these alterations are more likely to develop the disease. Alzheimer's caused by genetic alterations usually has a quick onset (middle age occurrence).

The precise causes of Alzheimer's disease are yet to be discovered. Scientists only know that the disease results from damages (usually permanent) to the brain. This disrupts the work of brain cells (neurons) and causes a series of toxic events. Neurons are damaged, and usually lose previous connections to each other and eventually die.

The damage generally begins in the area of the brain that controls memory. However, the actual process usually starts years before the first symptoms appear. The loss of neurons is a major characteristic of the disease and it soon spreads to other parts of the brain. Towards the later stages of the disease, the brain shrinks considerably.

Like most diseases related to autophagy, scientists believe that altered proteins play a major role in its occurrence. Beta-amyloid is a product of a larger protein. When these smaller protein fragments come together, they seem to have a toxic effect on the body's neurons and contribute to cell-to-cell communication disruption.

These clusters join together forming larger deposits called amyloid plaques. Proteins play a major role in the neurons' internal support and transport system. They help carry nutrients and other essential materials to the neurons. In Alzheimer's disease, proteins change shape and join together forming structures known as neurofibrillary tangles. These tangles disrupt the body's transport systems and are toxic to the cells.

Lifestyle and heart health

Recent studies have shown that heart disease and Alzheimer's disease share similar predisposing factors. These factors include:

-Lack of exercise/sedentary lifestyle,

-Smoking or continuous exposure to secondhand smoke,

-High blood pressure,

-High cholesterol,

-Poor management of type 2 diabetes.

It should be noted that many of these factors can equally reduce autophagy.

Living a healthy life can help reduce the chances of developing Alzheimer's disease. Studies have shown an association between mental engagement and the disease. People who engaged their brains more where less likely to develop it.

Alzheimer's disease and autophagy

Alzheimer's is not a preventable disease. However, a healthy lifestyle, especially one that promotes autophagy has proven to be very helpful. Elements of autophagy such as proper exercising, healthy diets (ketosis) and adequate sleep have proven to be very beneficial to patients. Many of the factors that help prevent the disease (as recommended by doctors/medical personnel) are similar to those that stimulate autophagy.

Autophagy equally helps prevent the formation of abnormal proteins. Scientists believe that these abnormal proteins are the cause/reason neurons get damaged. Autophagy also helps to correct malformed proteins.

Furthermore, autophagy is very effective in reducing the effect of the disease in ongoing sufferers/patients (palliative).

Prion disease

This is another neurodegenerative disease. However, Prion disease is an infectious neurodegenerative disorder. Prion disease is also known as transmissible spongiform encephalopathies (TSEs). It is a zoonotic disease (can affect humans and animals). Prions are infectious agents responsible for many fatal diseases.

Prions occur in different forms. Some examples of prions that occur in humans are kuru, Creutzfeldt–Jakob disease, Gerstmann–Sträussler–Scheinker syndrome and fatal familial insomnia. In animals, the most predominant prion is the scrapie disease. It is a zoonotic disease (transmissible to humans).

Prion diseases are known for their long incubation periods and central nervous system spongiosis. Prion spongiosis is associated with neuronal loss that alters the normal brain tissue structure. The disease has a quick onset of action and is classified as chronic. In severe cases prion can cause brain damage and even death. Symptoms may include dementia, convulsions, ataxia and behavioral changes.

Prion disease and autophagy

Prion diseases are characterized by spongiform degeneration. They induce the accumulation of misfolded and aggregated PrP (altered proteins) in the central nervous system. The symptoms are usually fatal (list of symptoms above) and neurodegeneration caused by this disease is severe. Recent studies have shown that autophagy vacuoles in neurons were frequently detected in neurodegenerative prion diseases.

Scientists consider that autophagy plays an important role in the elimination of pathological PrP (altered proteins) accumulated within neurons. Likewise, autophagy dysfunction in affected body neurons may result in the formation of spongiform changes.

Amyotrophic Lateral Sclerosis (ALS)

Amyotrophic Lateral Sclerosis (ALS) is a neurodegenerative disorder characterized by a gradual loss of motor neurons (both upper and lower motor neurons) in the central nervous system (C.N.S). The disorder is usually very severe and occurs mostly in elderly patients.

Statistically, Amyotrophic Lateral Sclerosis (ALS) is the most common motor neuron disorder in the world. It has an incidence rate of 2.7 per 100,000 and an age-of-onset varying between 50–65 years.

Symptoms include spasticity, quadriplegia and muscle atrophy. Patients usually die within 3-5 years (following onset of the disease). Normally, respiratory failure is the last complication to occur before death.

Available drugs include Riluzole, which prolongs survival by 2–3 months in some patients, and Radicava which helps to prevent decline in physical function. Like most neurodegenerative diseases, Amyotrophic Lateral Sclerosis has no cure.

The disease has two forms. These are the familial ALS (fALS) and sporadic ALS (sALS). sALS is the predominant form, comprising 90%–95% of the cases. sALS does not have any known genetic links. However, fALS affects 5%–10% of the cases (it has hereditary links).

Like many of its counterparts (neurodegenerative disorders), sclerosis exhibits the usual mislocalization of body proteins and the presence of cytoplasmic aggregates in motor neurons. This again points to an alteration in the body's protein metabolism.

Amyotrophic Lateral Sclerosis (ALS) and autophagy

An important pathological feature of ALS is the accumulation of insoluble protein aggregates in degenerating motor neurons and surrounding cells in the central nervous system.

These protein aggregates are typically formed by misfolded proteins that have been altered. The formation of misfolded protein aggregates is not totally pathological. It occurs naturally in the body (the body's cells continuously employ control mechanisms to either lyse the altered proteins to avoid aggregation or clear aggregates that have already formed).

Scientists believe that the persistence of these protein aggregates in diseased neurons suggests a disruption in autophagy. Autophagy is normally responsible for degrading/lysing altered proteins in the body. When autophagy is not functioning properly, this protein aggregate is causing harm to the body's motor neurons. Amyotrophic

Lateral Sclerosis (ALS) disease usually kicks off from here.

In both forms of Amyotrophic Lateral Sclerosis (familial ALS (fALS) and sporadic ALS (sALS)), immunofluorescence studies of post-mortem (dead) brain and spinal cord tissues have shown the presence of these proteins within aggregates.

Scientist believe that autophagy is the leading light (only chance of breakthrough) in respect to developing a lasting cure to the disease.

CHAPTER FIVE

How autophagy helps you build a stronger immune system

To effectively understand the numerous ways autophagy benefits the body, a clear understanding of the human immune system is required. The body cannot do without the human immune system. Without an immune system, the body would fall into the grasp of bacteria, viruses, parasites, and more. It is the human immune system that keeps us healthy and safe from various contaminants.

This immune system consists of a vast network of cells, tissues and organs. Its components (cells, tissues and organs) are constantly searching for pathogens. Once a pathogen is located, the body mounts an organized response against it.

The human immune system is spread around the body and is made up of different proteins, cells, tissues and organs. It can distinguish self from non-self (self refers to substances/particles/molecules that are homogenous/manufactured by the body, while non-self refers to those substances/particles/molecules that are foreign to the body). The latter are also called immunogenic substances.

When the human immune system encounters a pathogen (e.g. a virus or fungi), it mounts a response. This response is known as an immunogenic response. Below are a few important immune components.

White blood cells: also called leukocytes, white bloods cells patrol the body's blood vessels as well as the lymphatic system. Much like policemen, they patrol the nooks and crannies of the body, searching for pathogens. *(Autophagy boosts their effectiveness and enhances their actions).*

They can also trigger alarm bells. Once they encounter a pathogen, they send numerous messages/signals to other body cells. The storage of white blood cells is done in lymphoid organs. Examples of lymphoid organs are:

-*Thymus:* a gland located in the middle of the lungs and slightly beneath the neck.

-*Spleen:* the organ responsible for blood filtration, found in the abdomen.

-*Bone marrow:* Very important part of the body's hematopoietic system (blood producing system). The bone marrow produces both of the blood cells.

-*Lymph nodes:* small glands found in strategic places all throughout the human body. Lymph nodes around the body are linked together through the lymphatic vessels.

There are two main types of white blood cells (leukocytes). The first type is:

Phagocytes: They are also called antigen presenting cells (antigen presenting cells are cells that present antigens to the body for destruction). They surround and break down pathogens. There are several types, including:

- *Neutrophils:* these are the most abundant type of phagocyte. They attack bacteria and other pathogens.
- *Monocytes:* they are the largest phagocytes and are very effective antigen presenting cells.
- *Macrophages:* are also antigen presenting cells. They also remove dead and dying cells.
- *Mast cells:* they are multipurpose cells. They help to heal wounds and defend against pathogens.

The second type of white blood cells is the

lymphocytes.

They are also called memory cells. This is because they memorize previous history or attacks by pathogens.

Lymphocytes begin a cycle in the bone marrow. Those that stay in the bone marrow grow to become B cells, and those that leave the bone marrow (head to the thymus) are called the T cells. T lymphocytes and B lymphocytes have different functions:

B lymphocytes: produce antibodies and help alert the T lymphocytes.

T lymphocytes: are known as the action lymphocytes. They destroy compromised cells in the body. They equally help to alert other lymphocytes.

What is an immune response?

B lymphocytes secrete antibodies that attack and neutralize antigens. To successfully do this, the human immune system needs to be able to differentiate self-antigens from non-self-antigens. The body starts this process very early. It encodes all its internal cells (memorizes their details).

An antigen is any substance that can initiate/spark an immune response. Examples of antigens are bacteria, fungi, virus and toxins. Sometimes altered cells and old cells can become antigens too. All components of the human immune system work together to achieve immunity (combined effort/teamwork).

The importance of B lymphocytes

B lymphocytes are very important in the body's defense against antigens. Once B lymphocytes detect an antigen, they secrete antibodies. Antibodies are special proteins produced by the body. They are specific in action (specific antibodies lock up or attack specific antigens).

For example, a specific antibody is produced by the B lymphocytes in response to mycobacterium tuberculosis. This antibody would be different from that produced against pneumonia.

Antibodies are members of a big group of chemicals known as immunoglobulins.

Immunoglobulins play an important role in the body's defense against antigens. Examples of immunoglobulins are:

- Immunoglobulin G (IgG): marks microbes for easy recognition by body cells,
- IgM: attacks bacteria (major function),
- IgA: found in body fluids, such as tears as well as saliva, where it protects pathogens from entering the human body,
- IgE: guides the body from parasites. It is equally implicated in most allergies,
- IgD: initiates most body immune responses.

Antibodies do not kill or destroy antigens. Instead they lock antigens, and flag them off for destruction (destruction by phagocytes).

The importance of T lymphocytes

These are often regarded as the most important cells of the human immune system. They are divided into two: the normal T cells and the killer T cells.

Normal T cells: they direct the response given by the immune system. They interact with members of other cells (call them to the site of attack), stimulate B lymphocytes (to secret more antibodies) and draw a number of T-cells when necessary.

Killer T cells (also known as cytotoxic T lymphocytes): they are also known as fighter T-cells. They attack pathogens, especially viruses. They are the most competent cells in the body for this task. They recognize small concentrations of the virus on the surface of infected body cells. After recognition, they get rid of cells already infected.

Immunodeficiency

This is keenly discussed in modern medicine. Immunodeficiency arises when a component or components of the human immune system do not function. Immunodeficiency can result from a number of situations. These include obesity, age, malnutrition and alcoholism. AIDS is an example of an acquired immunodeficiency.

In some cases (very rare), immunodeficiency can be inherited (e.g. in chronic granulomatous disease where phagocytic function is impaired).

Autoimmunity

Autoimmune reactions are rare. In autoimmune conditions, the human immune system targets healthy body cells rather than immunogen/pathogens or faulty cells. In this condition (autoimmune disorder) they cannot distinguish self from non-self.

Autoimmune diseases include type 1 diabetes, celiac disease, Graves' disease and rheumatoid disease.

With this basic knowledge of the human immune system, the benefits of autophagy to the human immune system will be better understood. Recent experiments/research (using lab rats -MOUAU):

Resistance to disease (rats exposed to an autophagic lifestyle - Rats A)	Normal rats (not exposed to autophagy - Rats B)
Very high	Average
Immune cells - very active	Average

Rats A - Susceptibility to experimental pathogen (common flu)	Rats B - Susceptibility to experimental pathogen	Recovery rate of infected (Rats A)	Recovery rate of infected (Rats B)

30%	60%	High	Average
		Very fast	Much slower

This table creates a clearer picture of these benefits, although further details are given below.

Boosting the human immune system through autophagy

One of the major means of achieving autophagy (fasting) has proven to be one of the most effective ways of boosting immunity.

Recent research has shown that fasting for 72 hours induces immune system regeneration.

Fasting for 72 hours (3 days) can regenerate the entire immune system and reverse the damage done to the human immune system by chemotherapy.

Previously, fasting was regarded as bad or unhealthy. However, modern research results suggest that starving the body stimulates stem cells to produce new white blood cells, which defend the body in times of infection.

Recent research has shown that prolonged fasting can have a remarkable effect in promoting stem cell-based regeneration of the hematopoietic system. When the body is starved, it tries to save energy, and one of the things it can do to save energy is to recycle a lot of the immune cells that are damaged or redundant.

The findings from this research are revolutionary. With a renewed/boosted immune system, the chances of a long and healthy life are increased.

In fact, yogis and sages have done this in past times. Western medicine is only embracing it now.

How fasting stimulates the human immune system

Fasting is one of the pillars of autophagy. Prolonged fasting forces the body to utilize its stores of glucose, fat and ketones. It also breaks down a significant portion of lymphocytes/white blood cells (broken down for new cells to be generated).

In each fasting cycle there is a depletion of lymphocytes. This causes changes that stimulate stem cell-based regeneration of new immune system cells.

After fasting there is a reduction in the production of the enzyme PKA, a body hormone known to cause an increased risk of cancer and tumor growth. In addition, the human immune system of the subject (research done on animals) appeared to be boosted.

Prolonged fasting can reduce the harmful effects of chemotherapy

Prolonged fasting helps to protect the body from toxicity. This is an amazing development, especially for cancer patients who adopt chemotherapy as their treatment choice.

Chemotherapy remains one of the best ways to treat cancer. However, it causes significant collateral damage to the human immune system. The results obtained from this study suggest that fasting can reduce some of the harmful effects of chemotherapy.

The amazing benefits of fasting are not limited to the human immune system. Scientists believe these effects are applicable to many different conditions, systems and organs in the body.

Additional benefits of prolonged fasting

Scientists are beginning to discover more benefits of fasting. Below are some of these amazing benefits.

You will likely experience weight loss. First, you will lose weight because you lose water and stored products like glycogen. This is why increasing water consumption during prolonged fasting is important. In any case, depleting your glycogen levels will induce an artificial state of ketosis, turning the body into a fat burning machine.

Your body will "start to eat itself". This predictably leads to autophagy. Autophagy removes waste from the body and repairs any oxidative stress.

You brain activity increases with prolonged fasting. This makes sense when you think about it. When we were hunters and gatherers and we hadn't eaten for a few days, we needed to come up with new ideas in order to find more food: our ability to think critically has improved in these situations. Some research shows that ketosis benefits the brain, resulting in more brain-derived neurotrophic factor or BDNF.

Is prolonged fasting the same as intermittent fasting?

Intermittent fasting means submitting your body to a schedule of prolonged fasting (regulating your food intake over a period of time).

An individual may fast for 16 hours per day, only consuming food within an 8-hour window (eating between 11 am and 7 pm, fasting between 7 pm and 11 am the next day). Doing this repeatedly, or 5 days per week, means you are adopting an intermittent fasting schedule.

Prolonged fasting usually refers to fasting for a longer period. This is usually for about 2 days or more.

Autophagy and HIV

Recent research has shown that autophagy plays a role in preventing the replication and progression of the HIV virus. Autophagy was found to protect the small proportion of HIV-1 infected individuals who remain clinically stable for years in the absence of antiretroviral therapy. It boosts immunity (generates a constant supply of proteins to the immune cells). This gives them the needed boost and reinforcement they require to fight the disease.

Autophagy can be likened to an arms dealer (in the body) that supplies arms free of charge (to fight off HIV).

What is HIV

Before we discuss the amazing benefits of autophagy in respect to HIV, we will have a short rundown of the disease.

HIV is a virus that destroys (technically) the human immune system. The human immune system helps the body in its defense (from different pathogens - viruses, bacteria and opportunistic infections). Untreated, it infects and kills CD4 cells, which are a type of immune cell called T cells. Over time, HIV kills more CD4 cells. This makes the body prone to opportunistic infections (CD4 cells are very important defense cells).

As always, we shall discuss its mode of transmission, symptoms, diagnosis and treatment. Knowing the above is becoming more and more important nowadays.

HIV is transmitted through bodily fluids that include:

- blood,
- semen,
- vaginal and rectal fluids,
- breastmilk.

HIV can be transmitted or spread through different means. These include:

- through vaginal or anal sex (this is the most common route of transmission, especially among men who have sex with men),
- by sharing needles, syringes, and other items for injection drug use,
- by sharing tattoo equipment without sterilizing it between uses,

- during pregnancy, labor, or delivery from a woman to her baby,
- during breastfeeding,
- through "pre-mastication," or chewing a baby's food before feeding it to them,
- through exposure to the blood of a person living with HIV, such as through a needle stick.

The virus can also be transmitted through a blood transfusion or organ and tissue transplant. However, rigorous testing for the virus among blood, organ and tissue donors ensures that this is very rare in the United States.

It's theoretically possible to get infected through exposure to the blood of someone living with HIV, such as through a needle stick, but it is a rare occurrence for HIV to spread through:

- oral sex (only if there are bleeding gums or open sores in the person's mouth),

- being bitten by a person with HIV (only if the saliva is bloody or there are open sores in the person's mouth),
- contact between broken skin, wounds, or mucous membranes and the blood of someone living with HIV.

HIV is a lifelong condition and currently no cure is available, although many scientists are working hard to find one. However, with medical treatment (antiretroviral therapy) and a *healthy lifestyle (autophagy-based lifestyle),* it is possible to manage HIV and live forward with the virus.

HIV lowers the body's CD4 cell count, weakening the human immune system. A normal adult's CD4 count is 500 to 1,500 per cubic millimeter. An individual with a count below 200 is considered to have AIDS. **Research has shown that, when combined with an effective treatment, autophagy can help maintain the CD4 count in infected individuals.**

It's important to note that if an infected person is being treated and has a persistently undetectable viral load, it is virtually impossible to transmit the virus to another person.

Early symptoms of HIV can include:

- Night fever
- Body chills
- Swollen lymph nodes
- Body aches and pains
- Skin rash
- Sore throat
- Headache
- Nausea
- Running stomach

Prevention

The most common way of transmission (HIV) is through anal or vaginal sex without a condom. This risk can't be completely eliminated unless sex is avoided altogether. However, the risk can be lowered considerably by taking a few precautions. These precautions include:

- *Regular testing/checkups:* Knowing your status and that of those around you is very important.

Get tested for other sexually transmitted infections (STIs). If you test positive for one, you should get it treated immediately, because having an STI increases the risk of infection (contracting HIV).

- *Use condoms:* If you must have sex, especially with a partner you do not trust, you should learn the correct way to use condoms and use them every time you have sex, whether it's vaginal or anal intercourse. It's important to note that pre-seminal fluids (which come out before male ejaculation) can contain HIV.

- *Have only one partner:* This reduces the chances of getting infected. Promiscuity increases the chances.

Take your medications as directed if you have been infected. This lowers the risk of transmitting the virus or developing complications.

If you are sexually active, you should always ensure that you have condoms around.

Autophagy and HIV

Autophagy diets help reduce the effects of HIV on the body. It is not only limited to HIV (it applies to other diseases too). It also promotes healthy aging and reduces risk of heart disease, diabetes and cancer.

HIV is a chronic inflammatory condition, further stressing the already weakening immune system that accompanies aging. Dietary protein, trace minerals and antioxidant nutrients help to slow the rate of aging and can help prevent frailty.

Immune cell functions are sensitive to nutrition deficits. HIV infection alters gut microflora, impeding all nutrient absorption.

Nutrition is about providing materials needed by the body in its day to day operations. The balance between fats, proteins, fruits and carbs differs slightly from the normal autophagy diet.

An autophagy-based diet for someone with HIV should contain more fish and seafood and less meat than other diets. There should be liberal amounts of fruit and vegetables, including many wild greens in the diet. Whole grains such as cereals and sourdough bread are recommended. HIV patients should avoid pasta. Legumes, rich in magnesium, should be eaten almost daily. Fats should come from nuts, olives and olive oil. Dairy should be consumed more in the form of cheese than milk. Goat and sheep milk cheeses are recommended. Chemically, the diet should contain more selenium and glutathione, plus a healthier balance of omega-6 to omega-3 fats. The diet should equally be rich in antioxidants like vitamins C and E, plus resveratrol from red grapes/wine, and the anti-inflammatory oleuropein (obtained from olive oil).

Tips for Assembling a Healthy Autophagy Diet in HIV

-Choose healthy protein foods and eat them three times a day. *Unlike in the normal autophagy diet, HIV patients need more protein.*

The American Heart Association recommends two 4-ounce servings per week of oily fish. Statistically, very few people consume fish in a week, so a daily fish oil pill supplement should be considered. Up to 6 grams a day of fish oils have reduced triglyceride levels by almost 40% in an HIV population.

Research has shown that whey protein powder is a useful and cheap additive to a meal. It is often added to breakfast cereal or protein-fruit smoothies. Trials of whey protein in HIV populations' diets have shown that it can boost the human immune system and reverse glutathione (antioxidant enzyme) deficiency. Whey can also improve bone strength (prevent joint pain or other non-related conditions).

Consumed dairy products should be fat-free or low-fat.

-Add lots of vegetables to your diet for both lunch and dinner. Three cups a day should be the minimum amount to eat. This is needed in order to obtain Cretan-diet levels of minerals and phytochemicals. HIV-infected people consuming a dietary pattern that included a higher intake of vegetables, fruits and low-fat dairy foods usually develop a stronger and more effective immune system.

-Try eating fruit three times a day to increase glutathione and glutathione peroxidase levels. Eating fruit, including the traditional "apple-a-day," provides the body with water-soluble fiber (pectin). This aids the growth of beneficial gut flora, which lowers cholesterol levels, C-reactive protein levels and body percent fat.

-Nuts and seeds contain important oils that form cell membranes. You should try to eat a handful of nuts and one of seeds every day. **These oils help**

improve autophagy in the body (they help to rebuild the body and help boost the human immune system).

-Starches (carbohydrates) are the remaining part of fuel and food needs. Legumes, technically a protein-rich starch, are an important component of the HIV autophagy diet (however, the quantity of carbs should be reduced), providing fiber, plant protein and magnesium. Higher magnesium consumption is inversely related to cardiac and cancer mortality. More than half of the grains consumed should be whole grains. Whole grains are generally recommended as a carbohydrate source.

In addition to creating a diet that focuses on variety, nutrient density, and amounts, the calories from added sugars and saturated fats, along with sodium should be limited/reduced drastically.

Other healthy products to achieve autophagy (in HIV patients)

-Coconut oil: is a reliable autophagy inducer. Coconut oil is growing in popularity around the world. This is because of its endless benefits. Coconut oil has been found to be beneficial by doctors, weight loss experts, nutritionists and many other professionals. The benefits of coconut oil are so many that only a few can be discussed.

One of the major uses of coconut oil in modern times is in weight loss. Unlike many other oils or fats, coconut oil is made up of medium chain fatty acids. Medium chain fatty acids, as opposed to long chain fatty acids, are metabolized in the liver, before being broken down to ketone bodies. This simply implies that coconut oil supplies the body with a large amount of energy, thus restricting the urge and need to eat subsequently. This helps prevent the consumption of in-between meals that cause weight gain (excess weight gain for an HIV patient is not healthy).

Still on weight loss, coconut oil is also thermogenic. Thus, it stimulates the burning of fat in the body. Although coconut oil is not very aggressive in causing weight loss, it is very helpful when taken over a period of time and is very helpful in removing belly fat. Other benefits of coconut oil include improving cardiogenic function and overall health of the heart, treatment and palliative remedy for Alzheimer's disease, keeping the skin and hair healthy and radiant, maintaining dental health, improving the body's immunity, reducing inflammation thanks to its anti-inflammatory properties and improving gut health and digestion.

-Good wine: Yes! Who says HIV patients can't have some fun? From the olden times and until now, wines have remained very popular. They are classy and when prepared well give a quality luxurious taste. Wines are not just luxurious drinks (as most of us see them). They possess numerous health benefits. Some of these benefits include antioxidative properties which prevent cancer. Wine equally promotes

bone health, especially in elderly people, reduces the risk of stroke, has positive cardiogenic effect, reduces body cholesterol levels and helps to prevent diabetes. It is therefore safe to say that, when consumed adequately or in controlled quantities, wine can benefit the body greatly. *To cap it up, wine can equally induce autophagy (although mildly).*

Autophagy diets for the elderly (elderly people with HIV)

Reduced antioxidant activity coupled with mitochondrial damage underlie the faster rates of deterioration occurring in this population.

Common health conditions encountered in the elderly population include osteoporosis, vascular disease risk, sarcopenia, loss of cognitive function, fatigue/frailty and immune deficiency.

Subtle nutrient deficiencies can cause all of these problems. Using comprehensive nutrition therapy to treat HIV offers the opportunity to avoid increased pharmacologic burden in a population where side effects are pronounced.

The diet should contain fish, at least twice a week.

Vitamin supplements and natural calcium sources are usually not enough to strengthen weakening bones. In recent experiments, an algae-derived calcium was used, with strontium, boron, magnesium supplements, as well as vitamins D and K2 and the result was that osteoporosis was reversed in only 6-12 months in older populations (older HIV patients).

Safety measures can reduce falls at home and increased fitness levels can lower fracture rates. Equally, eating soft bones (biscuit bones) is very helpful, as it improves muscle action and helps improve body energy levels.

Consume lots of fruits and vegetables: An autophagy diet for elderly HIV patients should contain lots of vegetables and fruits. This would supply them with the necessary nutrients and vitamins needed to ward off infection.

Patients need to be reminded of the importance of positive lifestyle factors such as eating healthy, proper nutrition, and fitness in maintaining their health and improve the quality of their life while aging with HIV.

Food and *fitness education* can reduce complications in aged HIV population by 75% over two decades.

Multivitamin supplements boost the human immune system generally and are highly recommended for elderly HIV patients.

Autophagy based exercise

Exercise cannot control or fight HIV disease, but it is palliative and fights against many of the side effects of HIV disease or HIV medications. It can help you live a healthy life despite being infected with HIV.

What are the advantages of exercise?

Regular/daily exercise has the same advantages for people with HIV disease as it does for most people. Exercise can:

- Improve muscle condition
- Improve heart and lung performance
- Increase your energy level so you feel less tired
- Reduce stress
- Enhance the body's well-being
- Increase bone strength
- Reduce cholesterol levels
- Increase good (HDL) cholesterol
- Reduce body fat
- Improve appetite
- Improve sleep
- Reduce blood sugar levels

Exercise guidelines for people with HIV

A moderate exercise program will improve your body fitness and minimize health risks. At first, go slow and schedule exercise into your daily routines.

For starters, work up a schedule of at least 20 minutes, three times per week to the best of your abilities. This can lead to significant improvements in your fitness level and make you healthier. As your strength, stamina and energy increase, try to aim at 45 minutes to an hour, three to four times a week.

People with HIV can improve their body fitness levels through training like those who do not have HIV. However, people with HIV may find it difficult to continue because of fatigue.

Vary your routine so that you do not get bored. Find new ways to keep yourself stimulated to maintain your exercise program. Finding an exercise mate might help keep you motivated.

As your stamina might be reduced (following infection), it is very important that you work your way gradually. As little as 10 minutes is good enough until you build up to an hour. *Exercise induces autophagy and it brings all these benefits to HIV sufferers.*

Exercise with weights

Lifting weights is the most effective form of exercise (in respect to autophagy). Weight training (resistance exercise) is one of the best ways to increase lean body mass and bone density that may be lost through HIV disease. Working out three times a week for an hour should be enough if done properly. Doing weight training followed by 30 minutes of cardiovascular exercise may be the most effective way to improve body composition and keep your blood lipids and sugar down. Cardiovascular exercise means increasing oxygen supply to the body and heart rate while moving large muscle groups continuously for at least 30 minutes. Brisk walking, jogging, dancing, bicycling or swimming are all examples of cardiovascular exercise. Be creative about ways not to remain sedentary. The quality of your life depends on this!

An autophagy-based exercise program can improve lean body mass, reduce fat, stress, weakness and depression, improve strength, stamina and cardiovascular fitness. It can also boost the human immune system (make it perform better).

Autophagy and Tuberculosis

What is Tuberculosis?

Tuberculosis, also known as TB, is a very contagious infection, which most often affects the human lungs, and can be quickly spread to other parts of one's body, including the brain, without proper treatment. It is caused by mycobacterium tuberculosis.

In the 20's, tuberculosis was a leading cause of death worldwide. Today, a lot of prevalent TB cases are treated with antibiotics. However, recovery (cure) takes a longer amount of time, the treatment involving taking drugs for a period of six to twelve months.

In What Ways Can Tuberculosis Affect Your Body?

Getting infected doesn't automatically make you ill. The disease comes in two different forms:

-Latent TB: In this case, the virus is prevalent in your body, but it is in a constant battle with your immune system, which tries to prevent it from getting to other parts of your body. There would be no symptoms and the carrier would not be considered contagious. However, the disease still lives in the carrier's body and someday it might become active. If the carrier poses a high risk for the disease to become active, for instance people with HIV, the doctor would have you placed on antibiotics to reduce the chances of your TB becoming active. **People with a strong immune system and those who live a healthy lifestyle (autophagy lifestyle) usually fall in this**

category. Most times they are able to withstand the infection. The infection usually wears off with time.

-Active TB disease: The body is not able to control the disease. Those with active TB usually fall ill. More than 2/3 of adult cases of active TB result from the reactivation of a latent TB infection.

Symptoms of Tuberculosis

There aren't any symptoms for latent TB. You would need to get a skin or blood test to know if you're infected.

Signs of an active TB disease include:

- Persistent cough
- Chest pain
- Coughing up blood
- Weakness
- Night sweats
- Chills
- Fever

- Loss of appetite
- Weight loss

If you experience any of these symptoms, see your doctor to get tested.

Mode of transmission

The disease is airborne, just like catching a cold or getting hit by flu. Anything that involves fluid from any already infected person, like a quick cough, a sneeze, loud talks and laughter or any other thing that can cause saliva to leave the mouth, is one way the disease can be spread. This is due to the fact that saliva contains traces of the bacteria. Once you are unlucky enough to take in the bacteria (through any of the above), you can get infected.

Tuberculosis is considered very contagious but getting infected is not that easy. To get infected, you would be required to be around someone who is already infected for quite some time. This person still has to have a high level of bacilli load in their lungs. The need for proximity is one major reason it is quickly passed among people who spend time with each other.

Tuberculosis bacteria rarely survives on plane surfaces. Therefore, one cannot become a carrier simply by exchanging body contact or by partaking the food and drinks of someone who is already infected.

Risk factors

You can only get TB through contact with an infected person. Here are some factors that could increase your risk:

- A friend, co-worker or family member is infected.
- You live or have traveled to a TB endemic region like Russia, Africa, Eastern Europe, Asia, Latin America and the Caribbean.
- You are part of a group where TB is easily transmitted, or you work or live with someone who is. Members of this exposed

group include homeless people, HIV patients and IV drug users.

- You work or live in a hospital.

The role of an autophagic diet in recovery from tuberculosis

While the treatment of active tuberculosis is long term – up to a year of daily antibiotics – you can aid your recovery and help your body fight off the disease by making sure it gets an adequate nutrition. Your body needs healthy nutrients now more than ever.

People who are malnourished or underweight are more likely to get infected with tuberculosis and are also more susceptible to reinfection or relapse of TB after treatment. Malnutrition leads to decreased immunity, and your body needs to be as strong as possible to defend itself against tuberculosis bacteria.

Poor nutrition can actually encourage the persistence of tuberculosis, and this can lead to malnutrition. Therefore, to help your body fight TB, you have to feed it correctly.

To arm your body with the nutrients it needs to defeat tuberculosis and regain your strength and stamina, you need to eat a diet containing a variety of healthy foods (autophagy diet), such as:

- Vegetables, for their high iron and B-vitamin content.
- Reasonable quantity of carbohydrates, like whole wheat pastas, breads and cereals (in reduced quantity). In all autophagy diets carbohydrates are reduced.
- Colored vegetables such as carrots, peppers and squash. Fruits like tomatoes, blueberries and cherries. Colored vegetables are rich in antioxidants.
- Unsaturated fats like vegetable or olive oil instead of coconut oil or butter. Unsaturated fat has tremendous benefits (especially to tuberculosis patients).

Unsaturated fats are very useful, especially when they consign achieving autophagy.

Talk to your doctor about whether or not you have any nutrient deficiencies and if taking in daily multivitamins with minerals is necessary. A recent review of the limited studies done on supplements in patients with TB showed that high-calorie energy supplements helped underweight patients gain body weight, and that zinc, when taken with other micronutrients or with vitamin A, may offer nutritional help.

Avoid:

Generally, what is unhealthy remains unhealthy. Similarly, what is healthy remains healthy. Thus, a risk factor for tuberculosis can equally apply to several other diseases. Steps to be taken in order to limit these risks include:

- Avoiding smoking or tobacco.

- Avoiding alcohol. This can add to the risk of liver damage from some of the drugs used to treat your TB.
- Reducing consumption of coffee and other caffeinated drinks.
- Limiting refined carbohydrates like sugar, white breads and white rice (they limit autophagy - cellular regeneration).
- Avoid high-fat, high-cholesterol red meat and instead consume leaner protein sources like poultry, beans, tofu and fish.

Strive to give your body the nutrition it needs to maintain a healthy weight and build up body strength to destroy the tuberculosis bacteria and reduce your risk of a relapse. Eating a nutritious/healthy diet and staying away from unhealthy habits will help you feel better, faster.

Exercise

By now, you should know that exercise is one of the ways to achieve autophagy. People who are suffering from tuberculosis may have difficulty in performing physical exercise and being inactive during the lengthy treatment can make you feel weak. However, physical activity can speed recovery and help you manage your weight.

Recent research has shown that exercise can help the body fight the TB infection and not only speed your recovery but also improve your mood. If you have inactive TB, you can continue your normal exercise routines. You need a doctor's approval to perform or carry out any physical training if you have active TB. Moderate walking is a good way to start, especially if you are not used to exercise.

Start with short sessions, such as walking for 20 minutes. With time and frequency, your stamina will increase. You should walk as often as possible. As you build your stamina, you can increase your walking time gradually. Once active TB is no longer transmittable, if you feel well enough and your doctor approves, you should be able to return to your normal workout routines.

CHAPTER SIX

Autophagy and Cancer

Cancer causes cells to divide without control. This can cause tumors, damage to the body's immune system and other complications.

Cancer is a vast term. It describes the disease that results when cellular alterations induce the uncontrolled growth and division of cells.

Some types of cancer cause rapid cell multiplication, while others cause the body cells to grow and divide at a slower rate.

Certain forms of cancer can cause tumors while others, such as leukemia, do not.

The body's cells are specific in action. They have fixed lifespans. Cell death is a natural and beneficial phenomenon called apoptosis (cells die and are then replaced – autophagy).

A cell receives an order (to die) so that the body can replace it with a newer cell that functions better. Cancerous cells do not follow this order (are out of control).

As a result, they build up in the body, using oxygen and nutrients that would usually nourish other body cells. Cancerous cells can cause tumors, impair the human immune system and induce changes that prevent the body from functioning normally.

Cancerous cells may appear in one area, then spread via the lymph nodes to another part of the body.

Causes

Certain conditions or factors increase a person's chances of developing cancer. They include:

- Smoking
- Heavy alcohol consumption
- Obesity
- Sedentary lifestyle

- Malnutrition

Other causes of cancer are not preventable. Currently, the most important risk factor is age.

Genetic factors can equally add to the chances of developing cancer.

A person's genetic code controls the division of cells. Alterations in these genes can lead to faulty instructions, and cancer can result.

Genes also influence the body's protein production. Proteins carry most of the instructions for cellular growth and division.

Some genes alter proteins that would usually repair damaged cells. This can lead to cancer. If a person has a relative with these genes, the chances of that person developing cancer are higher.

Some genetic alterations occur after birth, and factors such as smoking and sun exposure can increase the risk.

Other alterations that can result in cancer take place in the chemical signals that determine how the body deploys or "expresses" specific genes.

Finally, a person can inherit predisposition for a type of cancer. Medically, this is called hereditary cancer syndrome. Inherited genetic mutations contribute to the development of about 5–10 percent of cancer cases.

Types

- Bladder
- Colon and rectal
- Endometrial
- Kidney
- Leukemia
- Liver
- Melanoma
- Non-Hodgkin's lymphoma
- Pancreatic
- Thyroid

Other forms are less common. According to the National Cancer Institute, there are over a hundred types of cancer.

Effect of autophagy on cancer (fasting)

The component of autophagy that affects cancer the most is fasting. Fasting may help with cancer treatment. There is growing proof supporting the role of fasting in both cancer treatment and prevention.

Recent research has shown that fasting helps fight cancer by lowering insulin resistance and levels of inflammation. Fasting may also reverse the effects of chronic body conditions such as obesity and type 2 diabetes, which are both risk factors for cancer.

Also, researchers believe that fasting makes cancer cells more responsive to treatment (especially chemotherapy) while protecting other cells. Fasting may also boost the human immune system to help fight or prevent its spread.

Improving insulin sensitivity

Fasting may help improve the effectiveness of chemotherapy.

Insulin is a hormone that allows cells to extract glucose from the blood and generate energy.

When food is consumed in excess, the cells in the body become less sensitive to insulin. This insulin resistance means that the cells respond to insulin signals slowly and sometimes they don't respond at all. This causes increased levels of glucose in the blood and higher fat storage.

When the food supply is scarce, the human body tries to conserve energy.

It achieves this by making cell membranes more sensitive to insulin. Cells can metabolize insulin more efficiently, removing glucose from the blood.

Better insulin sensitivity makes it difficult for cancer cells to grow or develop.

Reversing the chronic conditions

Recent research has also shown that conditions such as obesity and type 2 diabetes are risk factors for cancer. Both are linked to a higher risk of cancer and lower survival rate.

Modern research has also illustrated the effect of short-term fasting on type 2 diabetes. The participants in the study fasted for 24 hours two to three times per week.

After 4 months of fasting, the participants had a 20 percent reduction in weight and a 12 percent reduction in waist size.

Also, the participants no longer required insulin treatment after 2 months of this fasting pattern.

Improving quality of life during chemotherapy

Fasting may help reduce chemotherapy related complications.

Recent studies show that fasting improves people's response to chemotherapy because it does the following:

- promotes regeneration of all the body cells,
- protects blood from some of the harmful effects of chemotherapy,
- lessens the impact of side effects, such as fatigue, nausea, headaches and cramps.

A 2018 study showed that fasting can improve the quality of life in people undergoing chemotherapy for breast or ovarian cancer. The study was based on a 60-hour fasting period (about 36 hours before the start of chemotherapy).

The results show that those who fasted during chemotherapy reported higher tolerance to chemotherapy, fewer chemotherapy related complications and higher energy levels when compared with those who did not fast.

Boosting the human immune system to fight cancer

Fasting produces cancer-fighting effects in stem cells. Stem cells are very important in the body for their regenerative abilities.

Fasting for 2–4 days protects stem cells from some of the negative effects of chemotherapy on the human immune system.

Fasting also causes stem cells in the human immune system to regenerate.

This study shows that fasting not only limits damage to cells, it also replenishes the body.

White blood cells help the body fight infection and destroy cells that may cause disease. When white blood cell levels usually drop during chemotherapy, it affects the human immune system negatively, and the body might not be able to prevent infections.

The number of white blood cells in the blood decreases during fasting. However, when the fasting cycle concludes and the body receives food, white blood cell levels increase significantly. They almost double in number.

Cancer causes cells to divide without control. It also prevents them from dying naturally, following their normal cycle.

Genetic factors and lifestyle choices, such as smoking, can contribute to the development of cancer. Several components affect the ways the DNA communicates with cells and directs their division and death.

Treatments are constantly improving. Examples of current treatments include chemotherapy, radiation therapy and surgery. Some people benefit from more modern treatments, such as stem cell transplantation and precision medicine. However, most of these treatments are harsh and largely ineffective. Fasting (one of the pillars of autophagy) has yielded amazing results in cancer patients. Researchers believe that autophagy is the long-term solution to cancer.

Short and prolonged fasting periods have yielded amazing results in cancer treatment and prevention.

Stay young forever through autophagy

Aging is the process of becoming older. The term refers to human beings, most animals and fungi, whereas for example bacteria, perennial plants and some simple animals are technically biologically immortal. In a different light, aging can refer to single cells within an organism which have stopped dividing (cellular senescence) or to the population of a species (population aging).

In animals, aging can be described as the accumulation of changes over a particular period of time. These could be physical, psychological or social changes. For example, body movement or responsiveness may slow with age, while knowledge of world events and wisdom may increase. Aging is one of the most important risk factors in human diseases: of the roughly 150,000 people who die each day across the world, about two-thirds die from age-related causes.

Aging is a complex process characterized by the progressive failure of maintenance and repair pathways critical for cellular preservation, which results in a gradual accumulation of unwanted macromolecules and organelles. The accumulation of such oxidized, misfolded, cross-linked or aggregated molecules has negative effects on cellular homeostasis and on tissue and organ integrity. The defective molecules can alter homeostasis directly by interfering with the activity of functional molecules and organelles, which can cause further dysfunction. This progressive decline in cellular homeostasis leads to aging, disease and ultimately, to death. Although our understanding of the biology of aging has increased in recent times, the molecular events underlying this process have only recently begun to be explored. Interestingly, research in the last couple of decades focused on deciphering the molecular underpinnings of aging has shown that in many model organisms, the rate of aging can be controlled by altering conserved signaling pathways and processes, implying that the aging process itself may ultimately be receptive to therapeutic manipulation.

Dietary restriction and aging (intermittent fasting)

Dietary restriction, defined as the restriction of nutrients while avoiding malnutrition, is the most effective way of reducing aging. Dietary restriction was first observed to delay aging and disease in lab rats about a century ago. Since then, the effects of dietary restriction on aging has been studied greatly. Dietary restriction has been observed to extend the lifespan of yeast, invertebrates, fish, dogs, hamsters, mice and apes. Different molecular mechanisms have been proposed to improve the positive effects of dietary restriction on longevity, including insulin/IGF-1 and TOR signaling. However, it is currently unknown to what level lifespan extension resulting from dietary reduction is mediated by these nutrient-sensing pathways.

Aging (summary)

Aging results from the gradual decline in cellular repair and body mechanisms, which leads to an accumulation of unwanted cellular constituents and ultimately leads to the degeneration of tissues and organs. Decades of research have shown that the aging process is influenced by genetics and that many metabolic genes can influence aging by mechanisms still to be fully elucidated. Autophagy promotes cell maintenance by removing unwanted materials and by using recycled components as an alternative nutrient resource. This shows that autophagy aids longevity because an organism can recover more effectively from stress-induced cellular damage. Evidence that autophagy influences the aging process has been observed in different organisms, from yeast to multicellular organisms such as worms and flies.

CHAPTER SEVEN:
Autophagic Lifestyle

Autophagic meal plan

An autophagy-based lifestyle is key to living a healthy life and avoiding complications. Following an autophagy meal plan can help make sure that a person is getting their daily nutritional needs. It also gives you more options and can help in weight loss. We will now concentrate on autophagy meal plans.

We have done justice to exercise and fasting, but an autophagy meal plan can help an individual keep track of carbs and calories and make healthy eating more interesting by introducing some new ideas to the diet. No one plan will suit everyone. Each individual should work out their own meal plan with help from a doctor or dietitian.

Steps to take in creating an autophagy meal plan

- Balancing carbohydrate intake with activity levels and the use of insulin and other medications.
- Substituting calories with plenty of fiber to help manage blood sugar levels and reduce the risk of high cholesterol, weight gain, cardiovascular disease and other health issues.
- Reducing intake of processed carbohydrates and foods with added sugars (e.g. rice, spaghetti, cookies, etc.) which are more likely to cause a high sugar peak than whole grains and vegetables.
- Studying and understanding how dietary choices can impact your health (e.g. the fact that salt increases the risk of high blood pressure).
- Reducing and managing weight, as this can help a person manage the development of diseases and complications.
- Taking into account individual treatment plans, which will contain

recommendations from a doctor or dietitian.

Key points to note

- Having the right food measurement can help an individual monitor his or her food consumption more accurately.
- You can still enjoy a healthy, diverse diet that helps your body stay nourished.

As we noted earlier, this involves carefully:

- Balancing food consumption in order to meet the specific diet requirements,
- Getting appropriate measurement of portions,
- Creating meal plans.

Other factors to note when setting up a meal guide

- Take into account the daily consumption of carbs and calories.

- Take your time to determine the quantity of carbs that would meet your required daily consumption.
- Divide the quantity between the meals for the day.
- Always try to treat yourself. This can be done by doing a checklist of your favorite meals and including them in your dishes with respect to the carb requirements.
- Use resources available to you to fill out your daily meal schedule.
- Take note of your blood sugar levels to monitor the rate of results your meal guide is yielding.

Autophagy meal planning methods

These are some diabetes meal planning methods. Each has its peculiarities. It all depends on your targets or the state of your health.

Weight Management Method

There is without a doubt a link between diseases and body weight (obesity). Many people suffering from a disease may be aiming to lose weight or prevent weight gain. One method of achieving this is by "counting calories". The number of calories that a person needs each day will depend on factors such as: blood glucose targets, activity levels, height, sex, specific plans to lose, gain or maintain weight, the use of insulin and other medications, preferences, budget.

Dash Method

The DASH method is made up of the DASH diet, which focuses mainly on fruits, vegetables, whole grains, nuts and seeds. Other components include dairy products, poultry and fish that are low in fat or totally fat-free. This encourages people to avoid added salt, sugars, unhealthy fats, red meats and processed carbs. The dash diet has two targets: to reduce blood pressure levels and to help individuals lose weight and become fit.

Plate method

This method is growing in popularity. The plate method can help an individual get the right amount of each type of food. Getting the right nutritional contents/value from diets is important for everyone. The plate method uses the image of a standard 9-inch dinner plate to help people visualize nutritional balance as they plan their meals. It basically involves dividing your plate into sections, half (50%) for vegetables and fruits with the remaining half for protein, fat and carbohydrates. This more than meets the current recommended guidelines.

Carbohydrate swapping method

Although not a popular method, it is one way to manage blood sugar levels. You simply have to decide how many carbohydrates to consume each day and how to divide them between meals. You then create a replacement chart where you replace normal day-to-day carbohydrates (unhealthy carbs) with healthy ones. The carbohydrate chart ranks foods according to the number of carbs they contain, making it simpler to swap one type of food for another.

As always, seek advice from seasoned professionals. They might adjust your meal plan to suit your specific needs.

The Glycemic Index Method

The glycemic index (GI) ranks foods according to how quickly they raise blood sugar levels. Foods with high sugar loads increase blood sugar levels rapidly. Examples include sugars and other highly processed carbs. Foods with low scores contain none or few carbs, or they contain fiber, which the body does not absorb as quickly as processed carbs.

Listed below are some examples of carbohydrate-rich foods and their GI scores:

Foods considered low GI (having scores less than 55): pure stone-ground bread (especially pure wheat), unpeeled sweet potatoes and oats.

Benefits of an Autophagy Meal Plan

For clarification purposes we will briefly highlight the benefits of having an autophagy meal plan.

It helps save money

Meal planning helps you save money because you will know ahead of time what you will be cooking, and you will already have your grocery list ready to go. You will be able to plan meals around items you already have at home, which means you won't overspend on groceries, some of which will end up going bad and ultimately being tossed – the result of not following a list and buying too much. With meal planning, you buy what you need.

Knowing ahead of time what you will be cooking for the week will also save you from eating out and ordering fast-food. This doesn't only pertain to dinnertime. When you plan your meals and make sure to include leftovers for lunch, you will also save hundreds of dollars every month by not buying food near work.

Waste less time

An individual suffering from a disease may spend a lot of time on cooking homemade meals. More often than not, time is not only wasted on the cooking itself, but also while thinking about what to cook, making the grocery list and shopping for items. If you plan ahead to cook freezer-friendly meals in bulk, you will be able to save trips to the grocery store and time during busy weeknights. Saving time in the present is just as important as saving time in the future.

Waste Less

Statistics show that the average American throws away about 300 dollars' worth of food every year. Saving that money is a much better option. There is nothing more annoying than seeing food you bought with your hard-earned money wasted. By planning out all the meals you will be cooking, you ensure that no food gets wasted. As you prepare your meals, you will find this very rewarding and fulfilling.

Stress less

One of the most stressful aspects of daily living is planning meals. Thinking about these meals on a daily basis can be very frustrating. That is why having a meal plan in place can stop this unnecessary stress and allow you to slip easily into cooking time.

With an autophagy meal plan, you can expect to lower your stress levels. After following a meal plan, you gradually learn on the rope and you might soon find yourself making a new one in the future.

Lose weight (reduce sugar levels)

Home-cooked meals are healthier than eating out, because cooking at home gives you complete control over what you put into your body. Foods made in restaurants are great to indulge once in a while, but they are laden with sugar, sodium and fat. These are detrimental to the health of any diabetes sufferer.

But cooking in itself is not always easy. It is the meal planning part that keeps you motivated to continue cooking and stick to eating healthier. When you stick to a meal plan and enjoy more home-cooked meals, your body will start seeing results, whether you lose weight or feel physically and emotionally good overall.

Creates more options

An autophagy meal plan exposes you to a wider variety of healthy foods. This helps you have your cake and eat it. You stay healthy while eating delicious meals. In fact, if you don't plan meals, you are actually more likely to eat the same meals. This is simple logic. If you are familiar with making spaghetti and meat-stew, chances are you are going to make them over and over again to save time from thinking about what else to prepare. This could become very boring.

However, when planning meals, you can include new recipes. After all, they say that variety is the spice of life.

Learn portion control

Planning your own meals will allow you to see how much you are actually eating. This also prevents you from overeating at restaurants, which tend to serve a way bigger portion than you should actually be eating.

Eat healthy

When you are hungry and your blood sugar drops, you are more inclined to eat whatever you can get your hands on the fastest. This is why some of us settle for the closest fast-food joint with unhealthy options. Meal planning eliminates this issue when you have a balanced meal at your fingertips, filled with nutrient-dense food prepped and ready to go!

Many times, unhealthy foods are chosen because of convenience. Therefore, having an autophagy meal plan is a no brainer. *It is your gateway to staying healthy and enjoying your life.*

Meals that help you achieve autophagy

Vegetable omelets

Veggie omelets are filled with protein and fiber. All of the ingredients, from spices to eggs and veggies, are filled with a lot of nutrients, including lots of proteins and fiber. Its high fiber content makes it filling and satisfying. Vegetables are one of the healthiest ways to fuel the body for a morning full of productivity.

Ingredients:

- 1 teaspoon olive or coconut oil
- 1 tablespoon red bell pepper (shredded)
- 1 tablespoon sliced or chopped onion
- 1/4 cup sliced mushrooms
- Fresh spinach leaves
- 2 eggs (beaten)
- Water

- Pepper

Preparation:

Using an 8-inch nonstick skillet, gently heat oil over medium heat. Add the pepper, onion and mushrooms at once. Cook for about 3 minutes, stirring frequently, until onion is soft. Add the spinach and stir. Continue cooking and stirring until the spinach becomes tender. Transfer the vegetables from the pan to a plate.

In small bowl, beat the eggs together with water, salt and pepper with a fork or whisk until they form a smooth consistency. Reheat the skillet over medium heat. Quickly pour the egg mixture into the pan. Slide the pan back and forth rapidly over medium heat, stir with a wooden spoon to spread the eggs uniformly over the bottom of the pan as it hardens. Let it sit over mild heat for 30 seconds to lightly brown the bottom of the omelet. Try not to overcook. The omelet will continue to cook after folding.

Place the cooked vegetable mixture on one side of the omelet. Add cheese (optional) with a wooden spoon, fold the remaining half of the omelet over the vegetables. Gently slide out the mixture into your serving plate. Serve immediately.

Servings: 1

Nutritional values per serving:

Calories: 172 Kcal
Fat: 15.2 g
Carbohydrates: 5.7 g
Dietary Fiber: 1.7 g
Sugar: 3.4 g
Protein: 13.5 g

Ingredient Nutritional Analysis:

Olive oil

Olive oil protects the body against cognitive decline. Recent research has shown that the consumption of olive oil protects the brain and our learning ability.

It prevents the formation of amyloid-beta plaques in the brain. This is a classic marker of most neuro-degenerative diseases.

Olive oil prevents brain inflammation, but most importantly activates autophagy.

Harvested brain cells from rats fed on diets enriched with olive oil had increased levels of autophagy and reduced amyloidosis.

It is believed that olive oil is better than fruits and vegetables alone, and as an unsaturated vegetable fat it is healthier than saturated animal fats.

Researchers believe that an olive oil enriched diet improves working memory, spatial memory and learning abilities.

Olive oil increases autophagy activation, which can help reduce levels of amyloidosis.

This could be revolutionary. Autophagy activation in the brain will improve memory and synaptic integrity, and it can equally prevent the development of Alzheimer's disease.

Coconut oil

Though butter would make this dish tastier, coconut oil contains much less of both cholesterol and sodium than butter. This makes it healthier. Although coconut oil contains more calories, when used in little amounts, these calories are negligible.

Coconuts are high in naturally occurring unsaturated fat from short and long chain fatty acids.

These fatty acid chains are converted in the body into monolaurin, a useful compound that destroys a wide variety of pathogens. It helps fight common colds and viral infections, such as the flu.

Coconuts also contain the following essential nutrients that have tremendous benefits for the cell/tissue/body:

- Vitamin C
- Thiamin (vitamin B1)
- Folate
- Potassium
- Manganese
- Copper
- Selenium
- Iron
- Phosphorous
- Potassium

Coconut can be consumed in many different ways, and it can have numerous benefits for people with compromised immune systems and diabetes.

Coconut oil has recognized health properties when applied on the skin, but it can also have benefits when used in a diet.

Coconut oil should be used with caution. It has about 19 per cent more calories than the same amount of butter.

Coconut milk

Coconut milk is obtained from the coconut flesh. Coconut milk can come in two main forms:

- A thick form, called coco cream, that is used in rich sauces.
- A more fluid form, containing more water, that can be used instead of milk.

The more fluid form of coconut milk has the same number of calories as semi-skimmed milk. However, there are more calories in the thicker form (coco cream) and caution needs to be exercised in regard to portion sizes.

Coconut flour

Coconut flour is rich in fiber, which can prevent the risk of developing heart disease and can lower cholesterol levels.

It is low in dietary sugar compared to flours such as wheat. It is useful for people with diabetes as it helps them reduce blood glucose levels.

It is gluten free. This makes it a good option for people with celiac disease – an autoimmune disease that diabetes sufferers are more at risk of developing.

Additionally, coconut flour is a good source of protein, which keeps you full for longer and is valuable for cell regeneration (autophagy).

Coconut water

Coconut water is often regarded as the perfect hangover cure as it is naturally refreshing and full of minerals that can prevent nausea and/or vomiting.

Coconut water is the clear fluid found in young coconuts. It consists mostly of water. It contains very little fat and is very low in calories.

Eggs

The eggs account for almost all the cholesterol and sodium in the meal, but their cholesterol is the healthy type. It originates from Omega-3 fatty acids (especially fresh ones straight from the poultry). Eggs are also heavily responsible for making the meal filling. Eggs have been relied upon as a source of breakfast nutrients for centuries.

Vegetables and spices

The remaining ingredients in this omelet carry most of the nutrients in the meal (the seasoning and the vegetables). They contain lots of vitamin A and C, calcium and iron. The peppers contain most of the vitamin C. The spinach adds the potassium and is also a rich source of iron.

Yogurt breakfast pudding

Ingredients:

- 5-ounce bowl containing vanilla yogurt, one with considerably low fat
- 1/2 cup oats, go for the rolled ones
- A glass of milk
- 1/2 glass blended pineapple (juice pack)

- 2 teaspoons chia seeds
- 1/2 tablespoon fine vanilla
- 1/2 teaspoon cinnamon, preferably blended
- 3 tablespoons grated almonds
- Red apple properly chopped in fine pieces

Preparation:

Get a moderately sized bowl, pour in the yogurt, add the rolled oats, blended pineapple, half of glass of milk, teaspoons of chia seeds, fine vanilla and blended cinnamon. Stir well and pour into a container with a good lid. Cover appropriately and place in the refrigerator. Your content is perfect for consumption after a few hours.

Stir well before serving. Serve chilled. You can lace each serving with a spoon of almonds (optional).

Servings: 2

Nutritional values per serving:

Calories: 325 Kcal
Fat: 10.6g
Carbohydrates: 44.5g
Dietary Fiber: 7.6g
Sugar: 26.2g
Protein: 13.6g

Ingredient Nutritional Analysis:

Yogurt

Yogurt is without a doubt a great nutrient-dense breakfast option. If unsweetened (natural/without sugar), it is low in sugar and high in protein. This implies that it would not cause blood sugar to increase.

Fermented foods like yogurt contain good bacteria called probiotics. Probiotics help improve gut health. Although research on gut health is elementary, gut bacteria contributes greatly to the overall health of the body and can help resolve a number of health conditions, including obesity and high blood pressure.

Ongoing research shows that yogurt consumption might be associated with lower levels of glucose and insulin resistance in the body, together with lower systolic blood pressure. Nutritional analysis shows that yogurt, when included in a diet, can reduce the risk of type 2 diabetes in healthy and older adults. Another quality yogurt possesses is its low Glycemic Index (GI).

Yogurt and autophagy

High-fat diets cause obesity, leading to heart disease and autophagy imbalance.

Recent research showed the amazing effects of probiotics on high-fat induced obesity, heart disease and autophagy in the hearts of mice. Seven-week-old male mice were separated randomly into three equally sized experimental groups, namely normal diet and high-fat diet groups. Mice fed with a high-fat diet augmented with low to medium or increased doses of probiotic powders. These experiments were set up for a 9-week trial period. The structure of the left ventricle was analyzed using Masson's trichrome staining and immunohistochemistry staining. Key probiotics-related pathway substances were evaluated using western blotting. Abnormal myocardial structure and enlarged interstitial spaces were seen in HF hearts. These interstitial spaces were greatly reduced in mice provided with probiotics (yogurt) compared with HF hearts. HF was increased after probiotic supplementation was significantly decreased. This research has shown that oral administration of yogurt may prevent heart disease and cardiac hypertrophy. It also shows that yogurt aids the autophagy-signaling pathway in obese rats. These experiments are almost 100% bound to create the same effects in humans.

Coconut Berry Sunrise Smoothies

Smoothies are rich in nutrients. They contain a lot of fruits and vegetables. A smoothie can be a good way to consume a rich variety of foods. As mentioned before, these foods include fruits, vegetables and even fat, proteins and many others.

How to make a great smoothie:

-Include healthful fats: there are many good sources of healthful fats that can be used in smoothies, such as fats from avocado and chia seeds. Healthful fats can be good for the body. Fats play an important role in the body, and they can help reduce the speed at which sugar enters the blood. Thus, they can help reduce hunger or its onset. Examples of healthy fat sources are almond and peanut butter, chia seeds, avocado, raw pecans and raw walnuts. *It should be noted that no matter how healthy fats might seem, they should be taken in reasonable amounts.*

-Top up with protein: in a similar way as fat, protein offers many health benefits that are essential for the body. High-protein content helps to slow the absorption of food, and this reduces the rate at which sugar enters the bloodstream.

Protein can be animal or vegetable based. Vegetable based proteins are healthier. Adding high-protein ingredients to a smoothie can offer tremendous health benefits. Suitable proteins for smoothies include: plain unsweetened Greek yogurt, hemp and other seeds, almonds, pea protein and whey protein.

Furthermore, adding leafy greens like spinach can increase your smoothie's nutritional value.

-Include fiber: fiber can be soluble or insoluble. Insoluble fiber is harder. It takes the body more time to break down soluble fiber. Fiber takes longer to release its energy, reducing the risk of a glucose spike. Insoluble fiber boosts digestion and reduces the absorption of other foods in the gastrointestinal tract. Fiber creates satiety. These attributes can benefit a person with diabetes by reducing the risks of a blood sugar spike, an increase in cholesterol and weight gain. Through these ways, fiber can lower the chance of various complications related to most diseases, high

blood sugar and many other health conditions. High-fiber foods that can be included in a smoothie are: raspberries, oranges, nectarines, peaches and blueberries and vegetables such as spinach, grinded nuts (kale nuts) and seeds (chia seeds).

-Reduce Sugar: many foods used in preparing smoothies already have sugar in them. Processed foods often contain added sugar. Avoid using sugar (try to keep things as natural as possible). When choosing ingredients, take note of the following: honey and maple syrup contain reasonable amounts of sugar, ripe fruits contain more sugar than less ripe ones and milk contains lactose which is also a form of sugar. Spices are not exempted either. Spices such as cinnamon, nutmeg, ginger or turmeric fruits can be used in smoothies. Turmeric contains a natural source of sugar, as well as fiber. It is better to sweeten smoothies with natural ingredients rather than adding sugar/sweeteners. They are not good for the body.

-Reduce carbohydrate content: when making a smoothie, try to make sure you know the quantity of carbohydrates you are adding. Researchers recommend that people should look to include 45 grams or less of carbohydrates in a smoothie. Some examples of carbohydrates that can be added to smoothies are: banana, melon, blueberries, plain yogurt and granola. A healthy smoothie should contain spinach or other dark leafy vegetables. These contain fewer carbohydrates per serving and offer healthy nutritional benefits.

Using measuring cups, spoons and the diabetes exchange list is a good way to measure the quantity of carbohydrates to put in the smoothie. A medical professional (doctor/dietician) will advise on how many carbs a person should consume each day and at each meal. This will vary between individuals based on their height, weight, activity levels and medications.

About coconut berry sunrise smoothies

A rich blend of strawberries and blueberries gives this smoothie a vibrant purplish color. Coconut water, dairy-free vanilla yogurt and hemp seeds add a touch of nutty sweetness to give this smoothie bowl a refreshing natural taste.

Ingredients:

- 1 cup coconut water
- 1 cup coconut yogurt, vanilla flavored
- 2/3 cup fresh or frozen strawberries
- 1/2 cup fresh or slightly chilled blueberries
- 3 tablespoons hemp seeds or 2 tablespoons vanilla protein powder

Extra Ingredients:

- Sunrise Crunchy Cereal
- Dried coconut
- Fresh blackberries
- Cherries
- Blueberries

Preparation:

First, prepare the toppings for the smoothie bowl. Add dried coconut, fresh blackberries, cherries and blueberries to top this berry coconut smoothie bowl.

In a highspeed blender, add coconut water, dairy-free yogurt, frozen berries and hemp seeds. Blend on high until it has a fine texture. Shake the blender at intervals to ensure the mixture blends well (becomes homogeneous).

Pour the smoothie into a bowl and add the toppings (optional).

Notes:

Use frozen berries if you want a thick, frosty smoothie bowl. Choose fresh fruit if you desire a thinner consistency.

To get a different flavor, you can substitute the coconut water for vanilla almond milk.

Servings: 2

Nutritional values per serving:

Calories: 148 Kcal
Fat: 7.5g
Carbohydrates: 17.8g
Dietary Fiber: 5.6g
Sugar: 10.2g
Protein: 4.9g

Ingredient Nutritional Analysis:

Berries

Adding more richness to your diet in the form of berries is encouraged by many nutritionists. The amazing effect of berries against inflammation has been documented in many researches. Diets augmented with blueberries and strawberries have also been shown to increase behavior and cognitive functions in stressed young rats.

To analyze the amazing effects of berries on brain activity, specifically the ability of the brain to clear toxic waste, researchers fed mice a berry diet for 3 months and then studied their brains after irradiation. All the mice were fed berries 2 months before radiation and then divided into two groups. The mice in one group were evaluated after one and a half day of radiation and the others after 30 days.

After 30 days on berry diet, the rats experienced substantial protection from radiation compared to control.

The researchers studied neurochemical changes in the brain, particularly what is known as autophagy. Autophagy can regulate the synthesis, degradation and recycling of cellular components in the brain. It also helps the brain clear toxic wastes. Most brain disorders such as Alzheimer's and Parkinson's have shown an increased amount of toxic accumulation. Berries promote autophagy, the brain's natural maintenance mechanism, thereby reducing the toxic wastes.

Sweet potato, onion and turkey sausage hash

Sweet potato and turkey sausage hash is a great option for breakfast. It is gluten and dairy free. It is one of those few meals you can have for both breakfast and lunch. It is very easy to make and doesn't involve much processing.

Ingredients:

- 1/2 pound of turkey sausage hash
- 1 cup onion sliced
- 1/2 cup red bell pepper sliced
- 3 cups sweet potato sliced
- 1/4 tablespoon salt
- 1/4 teaspoon ground black pepper
- 1/4 teaspoon cinnamon
- 1/8 tablespoon cumin
- 1/8 teaspoon chili powder

Preparation:

Preheat a skillet over low heat.

Add the sausage to the pan. Break it up into small clumps.

Cook for about 6 minutes. Stop when the sausage turns brown. Remove the sausage from the skillet and place it on a plate.

Spray the skillet with a cooking spray and add the onion, bell pepper, sweet potato, salt, pepper, cinnamon, cumin and chili powder all at once. Stir until you achieve a good consistency.

Cook for another 5-8 minutes, stirring occasionally, until the sweet potatoes become soft.

Add in the sausage and stir to combine.

Finally, cook without stirring for 5 minutes. Serve hot.

Serving: 4

Nutritional values per serving:

Calories: 250 Kcal

Fat: 3.2g
Carbohydrates: 35.2g
Dietary Fiber: 6g
Sugar: 11.7g
Protein: 20.2g

Ingredient Nutritional Analysis:

Sweet potatoes

The sweet potato is gaining increased attention today, thanks in part to its low glycemic index (GI) rating. Sweet potatoes are ranked lower than white potatoes on the GI and they can help people with diabetes better manage their blood sugar levels.

Sweet potatoes are very rich in vitamins, including vitamin A which helps to keep the eyes healthy, vitamin C which helps the human immune system, iron which helps red blood cells to make oxygen and transport nutrients throughout the body. They are a great source of fiber, which can also stimulate the feeling of fullness. Even the roots of sweet potatoes are nutritious, although they are not frequently used in human diets/meals (they are used mostly in food for animals).

However, it should be noted that sweet potatoes are still carbohydrates and should be consumed in reduced quantities. Studies on rats (food and function research 2014) have proven that sweet potatoes help reduce high blood pressure, increase cardiovascular function while simultaneously supplying the body with antioxidants.

Ask a medical professional (dietician/doctor) for advice, as your health status may require a different approach.

Sweet potatoes and autophagy

Sweet potatoes are known to suppress endothelial senescence as well as to bring back cellular function in test rats. Researchers discovered that sweet potatoes aided autophagy to prevent that an increased level of glucose undoes endothelial senescence. Also, sweet potatoes prevented the prospects of endothelium getting older in rats with diabetes through the increase of autophagy. Reduction in autophagy led to a higher endothelial senescence, whereas increase in autophagy led to a lower level of senescence. In summary, sweet potatoes increased cellular autophagy, later on attenuated NLRP3 actions and also prevented endothelial senescence thereby reducing cardiovascular complications.

Sweet potatoes delay endothelial senescence by increasing autophagy!

Crispy breakfast pita with eggs

This very delicious meal is very light but surprisingly filling. It is easy to prepare and is a good option to consider when you want a quickie.

Ingredients:

- 6-8 slices of pita breads

- Olive oil
- 6 large eggs
- 3/4 cup mascarpone cheese
- Sliced zest of 1/2 large lemon
- Salt
- Freshly ground black pepper
- 3 tablespoons fresh lemon juice
- 3 packed cups arugula or baby spinach
- 8 oz thinly sliced prosciutto

Preparation:

Gently heat a grill pan over medium-high heat. Brush each side of your pita breads with 1/2 teaspoon olive oil and grill for about 2-3 minutes on each side, until they become crispy. Remove from the grill and cool slightly.

In a large skillet, heat 1 tablespoon of olive oil over low-medium heat. Crack the eggs directly into the pan and cook until the egg whites form (2-3 minutes).

Mix the mascarpone cheese, lemon zest, 1/2 teaspoon salt and 1/2 teaspoon pepper in a small bowl.

In another bowl (medium size) whisk together 3 tablespoons olive oil, the lemon juice, 1 teaspoon salt and 1/2 tablespoon of pepper until smooth. Add the arugula and toss until coated.

Spread each pita with 2 tablespoons of the mascarpone mixture. Divide the prosciutto into two (on top). Do the same to the arugula and place it on top of the prosciutto. Tactfully place a fried egg on top of each pita. Sprinkle the eggs with a pinch of salt and pepper and serve.

Servings: 6

Nutritional values per serving:

Calories: 391 Kcal
Fat: 16.6g
Carbohydrates: 36.3g
Dietary Fiber: 1.7g
Sugar: 1.7g

Protein: 23.5g

Ingredient Nutritional Analysis:

Eggs

Eggs are very nutritious. One large egg contains about half of gram of carbohydrates, which means you can avoid adding a lot of unnecessary sugar.

A full egg contains about 7 grams of protein. Eggs are equally rich in potassium, which helps to support nerve and muscle health. Potassium balances the effect of sodium in the body. Eggs equally promote the cardiovascular functions of the heart.

Furthermore, eggs have other healthy nutrients, such as lutein and choline, vitamin A (egg yolk) and calcium. Lutein protects you against disease, and choline improves the functioning of the brain. Egg yolks contain biotin, which is important for healthy hair, skin and nails (appendages), as well as insulin production. Eggs from pastured chickens are high in omega-3s, which are beneficial fats for people with diabetes.

Eggs contribute little to body fat. One large egg has only about 75 calories and 5 grams of fat, of which only a mere 1.6 grams are saturated fats. Eggs are complete meal agents and can be prepared in different ways to suit your tastes. They can be combined with a lot of foods to great effects (e.g. tomatoes, spinach or other vegetables). Although eggs are very healthy, they should be eaten with moderation.

Generally, one should limit egg consumption to three a week. If you only eat the egg whites, you can eat a little more (about 5). If you must fry your eggs, make sure you use unsaturated oils.

Boiled egg is a good high-protein snack. The protein will help keep you satisfied without affecting your blood sugar. Protein not only slows digestion, but it equally reduces glucose absorption. This is very helpful for the body.

JAIDA ELLISON

Crustless spinach and mushroom quiche

Ingredients:

- 1 tablespoon of olive oil
- 1 tablespoon of butter
- 1 lb fresh spinach leaves
- 1/4 cup yellow onion, chopped
- 2 cloves garlic minced
- 10 eggs (briskly mixed with a fork)
- 8 oz cremini mushrooms, rough chopped, stems removed
- 3 oz feta cheese crumbled
- Salt and pepper to taste

Preparation:

Heat your oven to about 350°F.

Roast the mushrooms by gradually tossing them with olive oil. Season with salt and pepper (little) to taste.

Spread the mushrooms on a baking sheet and allow to roast for about 25-30 minutes. Allow to cool enough, after which you chop.

In a medium sized skillet, dissolve the butter on low to medium heat.

Add your spinach and cook until it to begins to wilt.

Add the onion, then continue cooking, stirring periodically (every 1 minute) until the spinach is wilted and the onion has softened (3-5 minutes).

Add the garlic, then stir on low heat for about 1-2 minutes.

Remove from heat, then mix in the eggs, distributing the spinach and mushrooms evenly.

Pour into your prepared quiche dish and sprinkle with feta cheese.

Bake for 20 minutes or until set. Serve warm (steamy).

Servings: 6

Nutritional values per serving:

Calories: 210 Kcal
Fat: 14.9g
Carbohydrates: 6.2g
Dietary Fiber: 2g
Sugar: 2.3g
Protein: 14.5g

Ingredient Nutritional Analysis:

Mushrooms

Mushrooms contribute greatly to the body. They supply it with vital nutrients, can reduce/subside inflammation and are anti-cancerous. Here are some reasons mushrooms should be added to your diet.

They have anticancer and antiviral properties that have been used in Asia since the olden times. Mushrooms have immune properties and have recently been used in HIV treatment. They equally help reduce blood pressure.

Mushrooms help reduce body cholesterol, fight infections, reduce menopausal symptoms and fatigue.

Some species of mushrooms display anti-oxidative properties, reduce DNA damage, aid eyesight, fight colds, viral infections, reduce blood sugar (diabetes treatment) and much more.

Mushrooms and autophagy

Mushrooms induce autophagy in body cells to promote cell death. In a recent research, SUM-149 cells were treated with 1.0 mg/mL of mushrooms for 2h, 4h, 6h, 8h, 12h and 24h. To analyze autophagy effects on cell viability, cells were treated with 3-methyladenine (3-MA), chloroquine and PP242 with or without mushrooms for 1 day. Results showed that mushrooms affect the expression of autophagy-related molecules depending on treatment time.

Mushrooms increase the expression of autophagy proteins in body cells. Additionally, the autophagy inhibitors heightened cell viability after one day, while cancer cell viability decreased when mushrooms were added.

Thus, mushrooms induce autophagy, promoting cell death in body cells, as cancer cell viability is decreased, with an increase in pro-apoptotic protein expression when they are added in.

Lamb Stew

This is a very rich and delicious meal. You may be tempted to reserve it for special occasions. It is a household favorite. It has a rich protein content which makes it suitable for growing children and adolescents. Although its suitability cuts across age and growth needs, the lamb stew recipe is growing in popularity around the world.

Ingredients:

- 2 oz chopped bacon

- 3 oz lamb
- 1 tablespoon salt
- A handful of flour
- 1 bulb onion
- 1/2 teaspoon ground garlic
- 1 tablespoon tomato paste
- 1/2 teaspoon pepper
- 1/2 teaspoon dried thyme
- 2 bay leaves
- 3 oz nearly sliced potatoes
- 2 oz well grated carrot
- 1oz of thickly sliced mushrooms
- 2 cups vegetable stock

Preparation:

In a large pot, heat the chopped bacon over medium heat until it becomes golden brown and the fat is released. Transfer the bacon with a slotted spoon to a large plate.

While the bacon cooks, season your sliced lamb meat with 1/2 tablespoon of salt, pepper and 1/2 onion. Sprinkle the flour around the meat (1/4). Mix the flour and meat together. Cook the lamb under mild heat, and bacon grease over mild heat until it becomes brown (3-4 minutes per side), after which you place it together with the bacon.

Add sliced onion and heat gently for 2 minutes. Add garlic and heat gently for another minute, stirring constantly. Add thickly sliced mushrooms, bring to a simmer and cook 10 minutes uncovered. Preheat the oven at 325°F.

Return the bacon and lamb back to the pot then add 2 cups of broth, 1 tablespoon tomato paste, 1 teaspoon salt, 1/2 teaspoon pepper, 1/2 teaspoon dried thyme and 2 bay leaves. Add the potatoes and carrots then stir to combine (potatoes should be mostly submerged in liquid). Bring to a boil then cover with a lid and carefully transfer into the preheated oven at 325°F for 1 hour and 45 minutes. When cooked, potatoes will be easy to pierce, and the lamb will be very tender. To reduce fat content, spoon out any excess oil at the surface of the stew.

Serve with sugar free bread to soak up that broth which is loaded with amazing goodies.

Servings: 2

Nutritional values per serving:

Calories: 371 Kcal
Fat: 17.5g
Carbohydrates: 31.1g
Dietary Fiber: 5.6g
Sugar: 7.5g
Protein: 27g

Ingredient Nutritional Analysis:

Onions

Quercetin, a flavonoid found in onions, was reported to effectively inhibit 2-amino-1-methyl-6-phenylimidazo[4, 5-b]pyridine (PhIP) in food. Quercetin is converted into a novel compound 8-C-(E-phenylethenyl)quercetin(8-CEPQ). This compound can help prevent cancer. It is also known to promote autophagy.

Mozzarella and artichoke sauce

Although often considered a vegetable, artichokes are actually a type of thistle.

Ingredients:

- 3 oz mozzarella
- 2 oz artichoke
- 1 bulb of onions
- 1 tablespoon pepper
- 1/2 lb meat (preferably chicken) or fish
- A plate of chopped tomatoes
- A pinch of spices of choice

Preparation:

Fry the tomatoes with olive oil (add pepper, onions, spices of choice), preboil chicken with your spices of choice, pepper and salt. Mix everything together and after about 3 minutes add the artichokes and mozzarella. Serve warm or hot.

Servings: 2

Nutritional values per serving:

Calories: 328 Kcal
Fat: 13.6g
Carbohydrates: 15.4g
Dietary Fiber: 5.9g
Sugar: 4g
Protein: 38.3g

Ingredient Nutritional Analysis:

Artichokes

Artichokes are the real deal. They are low in fat while rich in fiber, vitamins, minerals and antioxidants. They are equally high in folate and vitamins C and K. They are also rich in important minerals such as magnesium, phosphorus, potassium and iron. To cap it all, they are rich in antioxidants as well.

Artichokes and autophagy

This vegetable has several benefits for our body. Artichokes contain inulin, a carbohydrate that is metabolized very slowly in our body, which is suitable for diabetics. Artichokes are very rich in fiber, and therefore help reduce blood sugar and control cholesterol levels. In addition, this vegetable can combat constipation.

The artichoke also contains cynarin. Cynarin stimulates bile secretion. Bile favors the digestion of fats and stops the retention of liquids (diuretic effect). The artichoke's caloric content is very low. It has less than 1% fat, and this is about 22 calories per 100 grams. Therefore, the weight loss ability of the artichoke is due to three reasons: its low-calorie content, its diuretic effect and its ability to digest fats and eliminate them. This makes artichokes very effective in respect to autophagy.

In addition to all that was listed, artichokes improve liver function as it works as a cleanser of the intestines, liver and kidneys.

Lower weight with artichoke water: artichoke water can be consumed three times a day. and at least 10 times a month. It can be used to treat obesity and also detoxify the body.

Herbed butter

Butter is classified under fats and oil. It is very beneficial for autophagy. Herbed butter not only stimulates autophagy, but it also contains nutrient rich herbs that stimulate the human immune system.

Ingredients:

You can make and prepare herbed butter out of any combination of your favorite herbs:

Cream the butter and herbs together and season with salt and pepper.

Preparation:

On a sheet of waxed paper, massage the butter into a log and roll up tightly. Fold the end flaps over to seal the butter.

Freeze. When set, slice off 1" pieces as needed and close the end.

Prepare ahead of time and freeze your butter, so it will be ready to go when you desire.

Serving size: 30g

Nutritional values per serving:

Calories: 210 Kcal
Fat: 23g
Protein: 0,3g
Carbohydrates: 0g
Fiber: 0g

Ingredient Nutritional Analysis:

Butter

Butter has long been a cause of controversy in the world of nutrition. Many nutritionists believe it increases cholesterol levels and clogs the arteries, while others think it can be a nutritious and flavorful addition to the diet. Fortunately, a lot of research has been conducted in recent years evaluating the potential health effects of butter. Recent research has shown that many of the old beliefs were wrong. Butter has a rich flavor and creamy texture. Although butter is high in calories and fat, it contains some very important nutrients. For example, butter is a good source of vitamin A, a soluble vitamin needed for good eyesight, smooth skin and immune function. It contains vitamin E, which improves heart health and serves as an antioxidant to protect the body against damage caused by molecules called free radicals. Butter also contains very small amounts of other nutrients. Examples include riboflavin, niacin, calcium, and phosphorus. It has a high calorie content. This means a very small quantity can provide the body with lots of energy. The idea behind using butter for weight loss is that by eating reduced amounts, you can induce weight loss through ketogenesis, one of the pillars of autophagy.

Pork carnitas

Ingredients:

- 2 tablespoons groundnut oil
- 2 kg of pork, cut into several large pieces
- 2 tablespoons salt
- 2 onions, chopped
- 1 clove garlic, crushed
- 4 teaspoons blended and already juiced lime
- 2 teaspoons finely blended chili
- A pinch of blended dry oregano
- 1 tablespoon blended cumin
- 14.5 oz chicken broth

Preparation:

Make the groundnut really hot, in an oven over low heat. Sprinkle your pork with a little salt and seasoning, then place the pork in the oven. Cook for about 5 minutes. Add all the other ingredients except the chicken broth. Incorporate your chicken broth after a little while and boil. Reduce the heat in the oven, safely place the cover and occasionally stir until your pork becomes tender. This will take about 1 hour.

After this, allow the oven to heat up until at least 300°F.

Move your pork to an already spread sheet. Do not throw away the liquid resulted from boiling your pork. Lace the pork in some of this liquid and add sauce to the mix.

Bake your pork until it becomes brown in the already heated up oven, normally a little over 20 minutes. Spray a little more liquid saved from before on the pork, every 5 minutes. Slice the meat as it turns brown.

Serve hot.

Servings: 8

Nutritional values per serving:

Calories: 440 Kcal
Fat: 13.5g
Carbohydrates: 5.8g
Dietary Fiber: 1g
Sugar: 2.2g
Protein: 70.1g

Ingredient Nutritional Analysis:

Garlic

Cancer is one of the most feared diseases in the modern world. To tackle it, humans have developed many high-technology therapies, such as chemotherapy, tomotherapy, targeted therapy and antibody therapy. However, all these therapies have their own adverse side effects. Therefore, recent research has been channeled towards natural food for complementary therapy. Naturally, they have less side effects.

Garlic is one of the most powerful foods. It has been used for many centuries for both culinary and medicinal purposes. Garlic induces cancer cell death by apoptosis, autophagy and necrosis. Studies have shown how natural foods regulate cell survival or death by autophagy in cancer cells. Many ongoing researches have shown that garlic not only induces apoptosis, but also autophagy in cancerous cells.

CONCLUSION

It has been a real journey. This book has intimately discussed autophagy. With the knowledge gained from its pages, every reader has now been armed with the greatest weapon to fight against ill health or disease.

This book was adapted to suit the needs of different individuals (people facing different conditions). Autophagy helps you manage your health properly. You can only get what you invest. This applies to business, and even your body. **When you see your body as an investment**, with the dividends now being good health and long life, you would have no problems in making these adaptations (changes to achieve autophagy).

We all know the popular saying **"garbage in and garbage out"**. If you eat unhealthily, you would most likely be unhealthy. But if you eat healthy, you would likely live a healthy and fulfilled life.

Best of all, eating healthy is not expensive. It simply requires you to adopt a healthy meal plan. If you properly follow the tips and steps provided in this book, in no distant time, you will reap the amazing benefits of autophagy.

This book is so rich with details that it allows you to have your cake and eat it (achieve autophagy with minimal stress). Oh yes! You will be exposed to life changing information, simplified to make execution easy.

OTHER BOOKS BY JAIDA ELLISON AVAILABLE ON AMAZON:

- Intermittent Fasting 16/8: Eat What You Love, Lose Weight, Increase Energy and Heal Your Body with this Lifestyle. Includes Delicious Fat Burning Recipes

Description:

Have you tried different diets among those in vogue and are you tired of not seeing results and/or have recurring weight gain relapses? Would you like a proven method that allows you to reach your ideal weight, increase your metabolism, and, at the same time, that helps you to be healthy and energetic?

You have certainly heard of intermittent fasting - the results it has brought to so many people in weight loss, and the benefits they have had in their health. This is demonstrated by scientific data and is not a trend of recent years, but fasting has always been practiced by us humans, since ancient times.

With this book, I want to provide you with a complete step-by-step guide on all aspects of intermittent fasting. In particular, I will dig deep into the method 16/8, which is the simplest and safest for those who are planning to fast for the first time and is, therefore, perfect for beginners. You will find that your body can become a fat-burning machine if you follow the right instructions and that intermittent fasting will give you the change you have always wanted.

Here are just some of the many concepts you will discover:

- Why intermittent fasting is a way of life and is, therefore, different from the usual diets
- What is the 16/8 method and the guidelines to follow it
- The benefits that you should expect
- How and when to exercise safely while fasting

- Answers to many questions that I am sure you have asked yourself about this topic
- Proven tips to make the most of and achieve success
- Delicious fat-burning recipes to boost weight loss
- And much, much more!

Perhaps you are undecided and hesitant because you do not know which program to follow, when and what to eat and drink, if this method is for you, at what time to fast; but you will receive all the information you need to start without worries and in the simplest possible way.

Link:
https://www.amazon.com/dp/B07XHSJW6V

- Keto Bread: Easy and Delicious Low Carb and Gluten-Free Bakery Recipes for Every Meal to Lose Weight, Burn Fat and Transform Your Body

Description:

Are you following the ketogenic diet and you miss the taste of bread while at the same time being tired of the usual foods?

Or do you want to start the ketogenic diet, but do not want to give up buns and bagels?

✓ If you're nodding your head, then you've come to the right place.

You will find:

- Tricks and a precious secret to making mouth-watering bakery products with keto and gluten-free ingredients, even without baking skills, that will allow you to avoid the most common mistakes that people make
- Which tools you will need to start baking your keto bread
- Which are the best low carb and gluten-free flours and sweeteners to use

- And which sweeteners you absolutely have to avoid to keep your carbohydrate level low instead
- Delicious recipes for Breadsticks, Buns, Bagels, Pizza, Toast, Muffins, Cookies... both sweet and savoury, perfect for every meal of your day
- Nutritional information in each recipe, so you do not have to stress out over macronutrient and calorie counting
- Easy to find and follow cooking time, portions, ingredients, and indications, even for a beginner

After reading this book, you will be able to:

- Surprise family and friends with astonishing and tasty keto recipes
- Discover the pleasure and saving of money in making homemade products
- Replace easily carbs in your diet and convert 'normal' recipes into keto recipes
- And much, much more!

Even if you think preparing your own baked goods takes a long time and you are always in a hurry, this book will surprise you, because you will find that you can make delicious recipes in a few minutes.

Even if you have tried to make keto bakery products in the past and these were neither tasty, nor looked good, or you have never cooked, this book will give you the pleasure of cooking.

Link:

https://www.amazon.com/dp/B07VXXD2GZ